Cell Cycle Control and Dysregulation Protocols

METHODS IN MOLECULAR BIOLOGY™

John M. Walker, SERIES EDITOR

METHODS IN MOLECULAR BIOLOGY™

Cell Cycle Control and Dysregulation Protocols

Cyclins, Cyclin-Dependent Kinases, and Other Factors

Edited by

Antonio Giordano

Sbarro Institute for Cancer Research and Molecular Medicine, Center for Biotechnology, College of Science and Technology, Temple University, Philadelphia, PA

Gaetano Romano

Department of Neurosurgery, Thomas Jefferson University, Philadelphia, PA

HUMANA PRESS 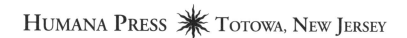 TOTOWA, NEW JERSEY

© 2004 Humana Press Inc.
999 Riverview Drive, Suite 208
Totowa, New Jersey 07512

humanapress.com

This publication is printed on acid-free paper. ∞
ANSI Z39.48-1984 (American Standards Institute)

Permanence of Paper for Printed Library Materials.

Production Editor: C. Tirpak

Cover design by Patricia F. Cleary.

Cover Illustration: From Fig. 1, Chapter 12, "The Transformed Phenotype," by Henry Hoff, Barbara Belletti, Hong Zhang, and Christian Sell.

For additional copies, pricing for bulk purchases, and/or information about other Humana titles, contact Humana at the above address or at any of the following numbers: Tel.: 973-256-1699; Fax: 973-256-8341; E-mail: humana@humanapr.com; or visit our Website: www.humanapress.com

E-ISBN 1-59259-822-6

Printed in the United States of America. 10 9 8 7 6 5 4 3 2 1

Library of Congress Cataloging-in-Publication Data   1004954696

Cell cycle control and dysregulation protocols: cyclins, cyclin-dependent kinases, and other factors/edited by Antonio Giordano and Gaetano Romano.

    p. ; cm. -- (Methods in molecular biology, ISSN 1064-3745 ; 285)

  Includes bibliographical references and index.

  ISBN 0-89603-949-8 (alk. paper)

  1. Cell cycle--Laboratory manuals. 2. Cyclin-dependent kinases--Laboratory manuals. 3. Cyclins--Laboratory manuals.

  [DNLM: 1. Cell Cycle Proteins--genetics. 2. Cyclin-Dependent Kinases. 3. DNA. 4. Fluorescent Antibody Technique. 5. Gene Expression. QU 55 C39265 2004] I. Giordano, Antonio, MD. II. Romano, Gaetano, 1959- III. Methods in molecular biology (Clifton, N.J.) ; v. 285.

  QH605.C4257 2004

  571.8'4--dc22

2004006931

Preface

Cell Cycle Control and Dysregulation Protocols focuses on emerging methodologies for studying the cell cycle, kinases, and kinase inhibitors. It addresses the issue of gene expression in vivo and in vitro, the analysis of cyclin-dependent kinase inhibitors, protein degradation mediated by the proteosome, the analysis of the transformed cell phenotype, and innovative techniques to detect apoptosis. Because there are already many manuals and protocols available, along with commercial kits and reagents, a variety of the more common techniques have not been included in our book.

The protocols described, based on rather sophisticated techniques for in vivo and in vitro studies, consist of molecular biology, biochemistry, and various types of immunoassays. Indeed, the authors have successfully accomplished an arduous task by presenting several topics in the simplest possible manner.

We are confident that *Cell Cycle Control and Dysregulation Protocols* will facilitate and optimize the work of practical scientists involved in researching the cell cycle. We greatly acknowledge the extraordinary contribution of the authors in writing this book.

Antonio Giordano
Gaetano Romano

Contents

Contributors

DOMENICO ALBINO • *Division of Population Science, Fox Chase Cancer Center, Philadelphia, PA*

ALFONSO BELLACOSA • *Division of Population Science, Fox Chase Cancer Center, Philadelphia, PA*

BARBARA BELLETTI • *Division of Experimental Oncology, Centro di Riferimento Oncologico, Aviano, Italy.*

BRIAN C. CHO • *Department of Cell Biology, University of Massachusetts Medical School, Worcester, MA*

CATERINA CINTI • *Institute of Organ Transplant and Immunocytology, Bologna Unit, National Council of Research (CNR), c/o IOR, Bologna, Italy*

PIER PAOLO CLAUDIO • *Sbarro Institute for Cancer Research and Molecular Medicine, Center for Biotechnology, College of Science and Technology, Temple University, Philadelphia, PA*

SALVATORE CORTELLINO • *Division of Population Science, Fox Chase Cancer Center, Philadelphia, PA*

MAJA DEMBIC • *Institute of Organ Transplant and Immunocytology, Bologna Unit, National Council of Research (CNR), c/o IOR, Bologna, Italy*

ANTONIO GIORDANO • *Sbarro Institute for Cancer Research and Molecular Medicine, Center for Biotechnology, College of Science and Technology, Temple University, Philadelphia, PA*

SORAYA E. GUTIERREZ • *Department of Cell Biology, University of Massachusetts Medical School, Worcester, MA*

KIMBERLY S. HARRINGTON • *Department of Cell Biology, University of Massachusetts Medical School, Worcester, MA*

HENRY HOFF • *Lankenau Institute for Medical Research, Wynnewood, PA*

HAYK HOVHANNISYAN • *Department of Cell Biology, University of Massachusetts Medical School, Worcester, MA*

AMJAD JAVED • *Department of Cell Biology, University of Massachusetts Medical School, Worcester, MA*

DARIO LA SALA • *Institute of Organ Transplant and Immunocytology, Bologna Unit, National Council of Research (CNR), c/o IOR; Department of Human Pathology and Oncology, University of Siena, Bologna, Italy*

CHRISTOPHER J. LENGNER • *Department of Cell Biology, University of Massachusetts Medical School, Worcester, MA*

JANE B. LIAN • *Department of Cell Biology, University of Massachusetts Medical School, Worcester, MA*

NADIR MARIO MARALDI • *Institute of Organ Transplant and Immunocytology, Bologna Unit, National Council of Research (CNR), Bologna, Italy; Laboratory of Cell Biology and Electron Microscopy, IOR, Department of Anatomical Sciences, University of Bologna, Bologna, Italy*

LUCIO MIELE • *Department of Biopharmaceutical Sciences and Cancer Center, University of Illinois at Chicago, Chicago, IL*

MARTIN MONTECINO • *Department of Cell Biology, University of Massachusetts Medical School, Worcester, MA*

SHIRWIN M. POCKWINSE • *Department of Cell Biology, University of Massachusetts Medical School, Worcester, MA*

JITESH PRATAP • *Department of Cell Biology, University of Massachusetts Medical School, Worcester, MA*

MASSIMO RICCIO • *Laboratory of Cell Biology and Electron Microscopy, IOR, Bologna, Italy*

GAETANO ROMANO • *Department of Neurosurgery, Thomas Jefferson University, Philadelphia, PA*

SPARTACO SANTI • *Institute of Organ Transplant and Immunocytology, Bologna Unit, National Council of Research (CNR), c/o IOR, Bologna, Italy*

CHRISTIAN SELL • *Lankenau Institute for Medical Research, Wynnewood, PA*

ADRIAN M. SENDEROWICZ • *Molecular Therapeutics Unit, Oral and Pharyngeal Cancer Branch, National Institute of Dental and Craniofacial Research, National Institutes of Health, Bethesda, MD*

LILIANA SOLIMANDO • *Laboratory of Cell Biology and Electron Microscopy, IOR, Institute of Histology and General Embryology, University of Bologna, Bologna, Italy*

GARY S. STEIN • *Department of Cell Biology, University of Massachusetts Medical School, Worcester, MA*

JANET L. STEIN • *Department of Cell Biology, University of Massachusetts Medical School, Worcester, MA*

TIZIANA TONINI • *Sbarro Institute for Cancer Research and Molecular Medicine, Center for Biotechnology, College of Science and Technology, Temple University, Philadelphia, PA*

CARMELA TRIMARCHI • *Institute of Neuroscience, National Council of Research (CNR), Pisa, Italy*

DAVID P. TURNER • *Division of Population Science, Fox Chase Cancer Center, Philadelphia, PA*

ANDRÉ J. VAN WIJNEN • *Department of Cell Biology, University of Massachusetts Medical School, Worcester, MA*

MARTYN K. WHITE • *Center for Neurovirology and Cancer Biology, Temple University College of Science and Technology, Philadelphia, PA*

ANTHONY T. YEUNG • *Division of Basic Science, Fox Chase Cancer Center, Philadelphia, PA*

SAYYED K. ZAIDI • *Department of Cell Biology, University of Massachusetts Medical School, Worcester, MA*

ALESSANDRA ZAMPARELLI • *Institute of Organ Transplant and Immunocytology, Bologna Unit, National Council of Research (CNR), c/o IOR, Bologna, Italy*

HONG ZHANG • *Lankenau Institute for Medical Research, Wynnewood, PA*

NICOLETTA ZINI • *Institute of Organ Transplant and Immunocytology, Bologna Unit, National Council of Research CNR), c/o IOR, Bologna, Italy*

I

ANALYSIS OF CYCLINS AND CYCLIN-DEPENDENT KINASES

1

The Biology of Cyclins and Cyclin-Dependent Protein Kinases

An Introduction

Lucio Miele

1. Introduction

In the 20 yr since the discovery of proteins whose levels oscillate during the cell cycle in marine invertebrate embryos (*1*), the study of cyclins and their cognate protein kinases has revealed a wealth of information on how eukaryotic cells control cyclical functions connected with cell proliferation and growth. The picture that has emerged from two decades of investigation is intricate and still incomplete. In the simplest possible model, cyclins are critical regulatory subunits of cyclin-dependent protein kinases (CDKs). When cyclin levels rise, they form stable complexes with CDKs, generating enzymatically active heterodimeric complexes. When cyclin levels fall, CDKs lose catalytic activity and are unable to phosphorylate their substrates. This simple model remains fundamentally valid, but it is now clear that the regulation of cyclin/CDKs is exquisitely complex throughout the cell cycle. Moreover, it is now widely recognized that cyclins and CDKs do much more than simply control cell cycle progression. The relatively simple mechanisms discovered in yeast cells, which have one G1 cyclin, one G2 cyclin, and a single CDK, are replaced in mammalian cells by a richly redundant molecular network, including multiple cyclins, CDKs, and regulatory pathways that cross-talk with a dizzying array of cell fate determination molecules. Thus, it is hardly surprising that initial hopes for quick discovery and therapeutic development of highly specific pharmacological inhibitors of cyclin/CDK complexes have not yet been fully realized. A few CDK inhibitors are currently in clinical trials, but their target specificity and their in vivo mechanisms of action remain incompletely understood. Having

From: *Methods in Molecular Biology, Vol. 285: Cell Cycle Control and Dysregulation Protocols*
Edited by: A. Giordano and G. Romano © Humana Press Inc., Totowa, NJ

said that, it has become apparent over the past 15 yr that the molecular circuitry of which cyclin/CDKs are focal switches is functionally altered in most neoplastic cells. A more complete understanding of how cyclins, CDKs, and their regulators are controlled in mammalian cells is highly likely to reveal therapeutic targets of genuine practical value. This chapter provides and introductory look at current knowledge, without attempting a complete overview of cyclin biology, which would be well beyond the scope of an individual article. Special emphasis is given to applications to cancer biology and therapy. The reader will be referred to recent reviews articles wherever appropriate.

2. G1 Cyclins: The G1 Restriction Point and the Link Between Growth Signals and Cell Cycle

2.1. G1 Cyclins and the G1 Restriction Point

The G1 interval of the cell cycle is the time that precedes the initiation of deoxyribonucleic acid (DNA) replication. Rapidly proliferating embryonic cells, which divide repeatedly without pause, do not have identifiable G1 intervals. Conversely, in most postnatal proliferative cells, the G1 interval is used to collect information about the surrounding environment (e.g., growth signals, nutrients) and make a decision as to whether to initiate DNA replication or not. The "point of no return" beyond which the cell is committed to a cycle of replication has been called "restriction point" and occurs late in G1 *(2)*. In general, antineoplastic agents that target cell proliferation can act either by preventing cells from crossing the restriction point (e.g., growth factor receptor tyrosine kinase inhibitors) and thus producing a cytostatic effect or by causing an ongoing replication cycle to abort during S, G2, or M, generally resulting in a cytotoxic effect, often mediated by apoptosis. Signals that influence the decision whether to replicate chromosomal DNA converge on G1 cyclins of the D family. There are two families of G1 cyclins, namely, D-cyclins (D1, D2, and D3) and E-cyclins (E1 and E2; **ref. 3** and *4*). All G1 cyclins can form complexes with CDKs 4, 6, and 2, thus potentially forming six different enzymatically active complexes. The tissue distribution of the various G1 cyclins is not uniform, with cyclins D2 and D3 more prominent in hematopoietic lineage cells, whereas cyclin D1 appears to be especially important in mammary epithelial cells and the nervous system. In the most widely accepted models, D-type cyclins form complexes with CDKs 4 or 6. Complex formation activates the CDK subunit by several mechanisms *(5)*:

1. A conformational change induced by cyclin binding allows access to the ATP binding site of the CDK subunit by removing the steric hindrance of the so-called "T-loop."
2. The same conformational change exposes a conserved Thr residue (Thr 160 in CDK2), which is phosphorylated by the cyclin/CDK-activating kinase (CAK) com-

plex *(6,7)*, which is itself a cyclin/CDK dimer (cyclin H/CDK7). This phosphorylation in turn causes a major increase in catalytic activity of the cyclin D/CDK complex.
3. Removal of inhibitory phosphoryl groups from two residues (Thr 14 and Tyr 15 in CDK2).

The main tyrosine kinase that catalyzes inhibitory phosphorylation of Tyr 15 is Wee1, whereas dual-specificity phosphatases that remove these groups belong to the CDC25 family *(8,9)*. Once activated, CDK4 and 6 phosphorylate "pocket" proteins Rb and its homologs p130/RB2 and p107. Rb, the best-known member of the family, is generally accepted to act as the main "brake" on the G1/S transition through its negative regulation of E2F transcription factors. Rb inhibits E2F-dependent transcription by physically binding to E2F and recruiting chromatin remodeling factors to E2F-responsive elements, including histone deacetylases and methylases and Swi/Snf complexes *(5,10,11)*. Rb phosphorylation by CDK4 and/or 6 partially relieves its inhibitory effect on E2F transcription factors and causes a conformational change in Rb, which exposes Ser 567, a CDK2 substrate. E2F then induce transcription of E-cyclins, which form complexes with CDK2. These complexes further phosphorylate Rb, thereby completely eliminating its inhibitory effect on E2F *(12)*. Once free of Rb control, E2F factors induce transcription of genes necessary for S-phase and DNA replication ensues *(13,14)*. Cyclin D-CDK4/6 complexes allow Rb phosphorylation by cyclin E/CDK2 in an additional way besides unmasking Ser 567. When cyclin D intracellular levels increase as a result of growth signals, the accumulation of cyclin D-CDK4/6 complexes "titrates" CDK inhibitors (CKI) of the cip/kip family (p21, p27, and p57). These CKIs do not inhibit cyclin D/CDK4/6 enzymes but rather form stable complexes with them and indeed stabilize the cyclin/CDK complexes *(15,16)*. When they are bound to cyclin D/CDK4/6, cip/kip family CKIs are not available to inhibit cyclin E-CDK2, which is thus indirectly activated as a consequence of increasing cyclin D concentration. G1 progression is also regulated by CKIs of the INK4 family, which specifically inhibit CDKs 4 and 6 *(17,18)*. For example, transforming growth factor-β often induces p15INK4B, which associates with CDKs 4 and 6 and promotes the release of cyclin D, which is then degraded *(19)*. This in turn causes redistribution of Cip/Kip proteins to CDK2, thus indirectly triggering inhibition of this kinase and contributing to G1 arrest *(3)*. Another INK4 family member, p16INK4A, is a potent tumor suppressor that accumulates as cells age and induces G1 arrest during senescence by a similar mechanism. Expression of p16 is commonly lost in transformed cells, often through promoter methylation, and is an often-crucial component of G1 checkpoint deactivation in transformed cells *(18,20,21)*. Low levels of p27Kip1 also often contribute to increased cyclin E/CDK2 activity in transformed cells *(19)*. Interestingly, the same genetic locus that encodes p16INK4A also encodes, in a different reading frame, another potent tumor suppressor, p19ARF. The latter provides a crucial link between the cell cycle and p53 by inactivating MDM2, the protein responsible for sequestration and degradation of p53. Thus, upregulation of p19ARF leads to p53 activation, which in turn triggers cell either cycle arrest or apoptosis depending on cellular context. Towards the end of a normal S-phase, E2F activity is extinguished by phosphorylation catalyzed by cyclin A/CDK2. This prevents the reinitiation of DNA synthesis and ensures that the genome is replicated only once (*see* **Subheading 3.**).

Abnormally persistent E2F activity induces p19ARF, and through it causes "emergency" p53 activation (**Fig. 1**). The outlines of this model for the regulation of G1/S progression (**Fig. 1**) are almost universally accepted. However, there is still disagreement on many details. For instance, this model implies that cyclin E/CDK2 complexes are indispensable for entry into S-phase. However, recent evidence suggests that this is not always the case and CDK2 is dispensable for cell replication in transformed cells *(22)*. This poses an obvious problem for drug development because even highly specific inhibitors of CDK2 may not have the desired cytostatic effect in vivo. It is quite possible that in the absence of CDK2, other G1 CDKs can replace its functions, at least in neoplastic cells. This illustrates a fundamental problem in cell cycle studies in mammalian cells, namely, the importance of functional redundancy. With at least five G1 cyclins and three G1 kinases, the machinery that catalyzes Rb phosphorylation is highly redundant, and the lack of an individual component is not necessarily going to have drastic consequences. The redundancy picture becomes even more complicated if we recall that there are at least 3 Rb-family "pocket" proteins, and six E2F family transcription factors with two DP heterodimerization partners *(14)*. This extensively redundant circuitry poses a formidable challenge for those who are attempting to manipulate the cell cycle machinery pharmacologically.

2.2. Regulation of Expression and Activity of G1 Cyclins

Despite this apparently hopeless complexity, several facts are solidly established. D-type cyclins have the unique function of acting as a link between extracellular proliferation and growth signals and the cell cycle machinery. The expression of D-cyclins is under transcriptional control that responds to several growth factor-activated cascades, unlike expression of E, A, or B cyclins. Transcription factors that induce cyclin D expression include signal transducers and activators of transcription (STATs), nuclear factor (NF)-κB, Ets, some varieties of activator protein (AP)-1, including JunB but not c-Jun and TCF-LEF *(5)*. These, in turn, are activated by various hematopoietic growth factors and cytokines (STAT, NF-κB), *Ras*-MEK–ERK-mediated signals (ets, AP-1), Wnt-β-catenin (TCF-LEF), and Notch receptors (presumably acting via NF-κB; ref. *23*). Conversely, E2F and PPARγ transcription factors inhibit cyclin D expression *(5)*. Intracellular levels of cyclin D expression are also controlled post-transcriptionally by proteasome-mediated proteolysis after ubiquitination. Free cyclin D1, for example, has a short half-life (approx 20 min), because it is ubiquitinated and targeted for degradation by the Skp1/CDC53/Fbox (SCF) complex through its component Cul-1 *(24)*. This process is promoted by cyclin D phosphorylation catalyzed by glycogen synthase kinase 3β (GSK3β) *(25)*. The latter is inhibited by AKT *(26)* and by Wnt mediator Disheveled *(27,28)*. Thus,

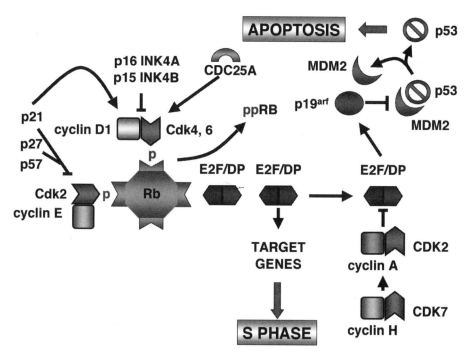

Fig. 1. Regulation of the G1-S transition. Rb is the primary "brake" at the G1 restriction point. Cyclin D/CDK4/6 complexes phosphorylate Rb and make it accessible to further phosphorylation by cyclin E/CDK2. G1 Cyclin/CDK complexes are activated by protein phosphatase CDC25A, which removes inhibitory phosphates at Thr 14 and Tyr 15. Cip-Kip family CKIs p21, p27, and p57 form stable, noninhibitory complexes with cyclin D/CDKs and are thus prevented from inhibiting CDK2. INK4 family CKIs p14 and p16 specifically inhibit CDK4/6, releasing Cip-Kip family CKIs, which are then free to inhibit CDK2. Once fully phosphorylated, Rb becomes unable to inhibit heterodimeric transcription factors E2F/DP (E2F for short). E2F activation induces expression of genes necessary for entry into S phase. In late S-phase, cyclin A/CDK2, which is in turn activated by CAK (cyclin H/CDK7) phosphorylates and inactivates E2F. This ensures that DNA synthesis is not re-initiated and allows exit from S-phase. If cyclin A/CDK2 fails to inactivate E2F, persistent E2F activity induces expression of p19arf (from a different reading frame of the INK4A gene). The latter prevents p53 degradation by MDM2, thereby allowing accumulation of p53 and triggering apoptosis. Thus, continued E2F activity beyond late S-phase can cause cell death. Pointed arrows indicate stimulation, while flat-tipped arrows indicate inhibition.

survival/proliferation signals conveyed by PI3 kinase/AKT pathway or the Wnt/Frizzled/Dishevelled pathway stabilize cyclin D via inhibition of GSK3β. **Figure 2** depicts a simplified scheme of the regulation cyclin D1 levels by mitogens and growth factors.

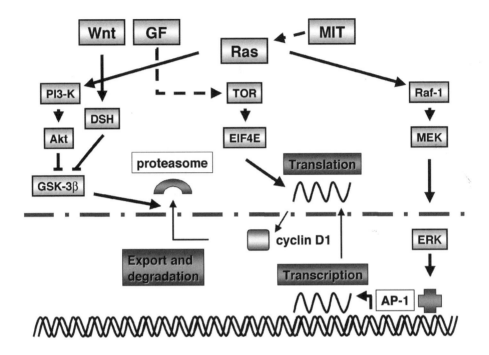

Fig. 2. Cyclin D1 levels are regulated by mitogens and growth factors through transcriptional and post-transcriptional mechanisms. Cyclin D1 provides a crucial link between extracellular stimuli such as mitogens and growth factors and the cell cycle machinery. The expression of cyclin D1 mRNA is controlled at the transcriptional level by numerous extracellularly regulated transcription factors. In this example, mitogens (MIT) acting through *Ras* activate heterodimeric transcription factor AP-1 via the MEK-ERK pathway, leading to cyclin D1 transcription. Not all forms of AP-1 induce cyclin D1. Growth factors (GF), acting through TOR and initiation factor EIF4E, enhance the rate of translation of many mRNAs, including that of cyclin D1. Finally, cyclin D1 (as a complex with CDK4) is exported from the nucleus and degraded through a proteasome-mediated mechanism. GSK-3β stimulates this process. Pathways acting through PI3 kinase-AKT, including *Ras*, and the Wnt-Disheveled (DSH) pathway, inhibit GSK-3β leading to cyclin D1 accumulation. Pointed arrows indicate stimulation or migration (e.g., outside the nucleus), while flat-tipped arrows indicate inhibition.

2.3. Beyond G1: Additional Roles of G1 Cyclins

Consistent with their role as transducers of growth signals, D-type cyclins have additional functions besides Rb phosphorylation. First, they somehow activate the process of cell growth, that is, the process through which cells increase in mass. The role of cyclin D-CDK4 in cell growth has been revealed by *Drosophila, Caenorhabditis elegans*, and *Arabidopsis* studies. In these organisms, defects of either cyclin D or CDK4 result in stunted cell growth *(5)*. Intuitively, it is clear that to proliferate, a cell has to increase in mass first. Thus, it is not surprising that a key early mediator of cell proliferation can also activate cell growth. Cell growth signals are largely transduced via the target of rapamycin (TOR) proteins *(29–31)*. TOR, in cooperation with the PI3-kinase/AKT pathway, increase the rate of mRNA translation by activating the p70S6K ribosomal protein kinase and blocking the translation inhibitor 4E-BP1, which inactivates initiation factor EIF-4E. Thus, the end result of TOR activation is an increased rate of protein synthesis. This includes enhanced translation of cyclin D1 (**Fig. 2**). The latter induces cell growth by poorly defined mechanisms *(5,32)*.

D-type cyclins, especially cyclin D1, have additional functions that are not mediated by interaction with CDKs 4 or 6. Specific interactions of cyclin D1 with a number of transcription factors have been documented. These result in either transcriptional activation or inhibition depending on the target. Specifically, cyclin D1 interacts with the estrogen receptor (ER), mediating an increase in ER-dependent transcription that can be independent of ligand. Immunodetectable cyclin D1 can be found in association with ER in normal and malignant breast cells *(33,34)*. Conversely, cyclin D1 represses the transcriptional activity of a number of other factors, including STAT3, Sp1, DMP1, thyroid hormone receptors, and androgen receptors *(5)*. Because STAT3 and Sp1 regulate cyclin D1 transcription, the possibility of both positive and negative feedback mechanisms exists. In addition, binding of cyclin D1 with a variety of transcriptional coregulators and general (i.e., nongene specific) transcription factors has been described. Known binding partners include transcriptional co-activators of the p160 family such as NcoA/SRC1a, AIB-1, and GRIP-1 that are involved in steroid receptor activities. It appears that the activating effects of cyclin D1 on ER are mediated by p160 binding. Conversely, cyclin–D1/CDK4 complexes can block the activity of myogenic transcription factor MEF by binding its p160 co-activator GRIP1 *(5)*. Another cyclin D1 binding partner is histone acetyltransferase P/CAF *(35)*. Titration of P/CAF may explain the inhibitory activity of cyclin D1 on the androgen receptor. At least under overexpression conditions, cyclin D1 also interacts with histone deacetylase HDAC3 *(36)*. It is unclear whether this interaction is direct or mediated. Thus, the potential exists that cyclin D1, alone or in a complex with CDK4, may regulate the acetylation and/or deacetylation not only of chromatin histones, but also of other targets of the acetylase/deacetylase enzymes. Besides transcriptional co-factors and histone acetylases/deacetylases, cyclin D1/CDK4 has been reported to interact with the general transcriptional machinery, specifically, with TATA-binding protein component TAFII250 *(5,37)*. This raises the issue of whether CDK4 kinase activity is required for the function of the transcriptional–preinitiation complex under physiological conditions. An additional issue is whether any or all of the putative transcriptional effects of cyclin D1 may require the co-association with p21cip1/waf1, which is for the most part found in association with cyclin–D/CDK complexes. Whether these transcriptional effects of cyclin D1 occur under physiological conditions or are consequences of cyclin D1 overexpression, such as is commonly observed in transformed cells, remains an open question. In this regard, it is important to recall that D1-deficient mice are viable, though they show abnormalities in mammary epithelial, retina and Schwann cells *(5,38,39)*. Additionally, cyclin E "knock-in" can rescue the phenotype of cyclin D1-deficient mice *(40)*. This suggests that either other cyclins (D2, D3, E) can replace cyclin D1 in both its cell cycle-related and transcriptional functions, or that the transcriptional functions of cyclin D1 are redundant under physiological conditions. However, this does not necessarily mean that the same is true in those neoplastic cells that overexpress cyclin D1. Cyclin E has been also reported to have transcriptional effects, but these are distinct from those of D-type cyclins. For example, cyclin E/CDK2 can activate transcription factor NPAT, which in turn is a CDK2 substrate and contributes to its effect on cell cycle progression *(41,42)*.

3. Cyclin A: Driving S-Phase, But Only Once Per Cycle

Cyclin A starts to accumulate during S phase, and is destroyed during mitosis before metaphase by proteasome-mediated cleavage *(43)*. E2F transcription factors induce cyclin A expression, after they are relieved from Rb-mediated inhibition by the sequential action of G1–cyclin/CDK complexes. This assures that cyclin A synthesis follows passage through the G1 checkpoint. The main demonstrated functions of cyclin A are to promote DNA replication while at the same time assuring that only one round of genome replication takes place at each cell cycle. Cyclin A forms a complex with CDK2 and phosphorylates a range of substrates, including components of the DNA replication machinery such as CDC6 *(43)*. Additionally and perhaps more importantly, cyclin A/CDK2 phosphorylates E2F-1/DP complexes, inactivating them *(43,44)*. This prevents a reinitiation of DNA replication and assures that the genome is replicated only once at each S phase. Failure of cyclin A/CDK2 to inactivate E2F results in inappropriately persistent E2F activity, which triggers apoptosis, in large part via p19arf and p53 (*see* **Subheading 2.1.** and **Figure 1**). This makes cyclin A/CDK2 a potentially important therapeutic target, and inhibition of cyclin A/CDK2 may participate in the mechanism of action of CDK inhibitors such as flavopiridol. In addition to its functions in S phase, cyclin A is thought to play a poorly defined role in mitosis, at least until metaphase. Cyclin A can associate with CDK1, as does cyclin B (*see* **subheading 4.**) and in *Drosophila,* it can rescue the effects of cyclin B loss *(45)*. This further underscores the biological significance of functional redundancy between cyclins and their kinase partners.

4. Cyclin B/Cdk1: The Gatekeeper to Mitosis

Drugs that inhibit or arrest mitosis have been found empirically to be among the most effective chemotherapeutic agents available. Not surprisingly, the mitotic machinery remains an area of enormous basic and translational scientific interest. Fortunately, the components of this machinery are highly conserved among eukaryotic cells, and this has allowed considerable insights to be gained from the study of simple organisms such as yeast or invertebrates. The cyclin–B/CDK1 complex is critical for the onset of mitosis in all eukaryotic cells. The kinase subunit was originally known as cdc2 in fission yeast and cdc28 in budding yeast respectively. As is the case for G1–cyclin/CDK complexes, cyclin B/CDK1 is regulated by both activating and inhibitory phosphorylations. Specifically, CDK1 Tyr 15 phosphorylation by Wee1 *(7)* or Myt1 and Thr14 phosphorylation by Myt1 *(45,46)* inhibit the activation of the complex, whereas Thr161 phosphorylation enhances its activity by allowing a stable association with cyclin B. The complex is activated at the onset of mitosis, largely through a combination of Wee1 inactivation and dephosphorylation catalyzed by CDC25C protein phosphatase *(45)*. During a normal cell cycle, negative regulation of cyclin B/CDK1 prevents premature mitotic entry prior to completion of S phase. The inhibitory actions of the two kinases Wee1 and Myt1 allow the accumulation of a large reserve of inactive cyclin–B/Cdk1 complexes during G2 phase, before commitment to mitosis. The abrupt dephosphorylation of Tyr15 and Thr14 by dual-specificity phosphatase CDC25C creates a spike in cyclin B/CDK1. Once activated, cyclin B/CDK1 phosphorylates and inactivates its own inhibitors Wee1 and Myt1, whereas it also phosphorylates and activates its own activator CDC25C. Thus, a small increase in cyclin B/CDK1 activity can produce a positive feedback cascade that causes a rapid and massive increase in overall CDK1 activity (**Fig. 3**). Active cyclin B/CDK1 a range of substrates that promote entry into mitosis and progression through mitosis. Cdk1 substrates include nuclear lamins, kinesin-related motors and other microtubule-binding proteins, condensins, and Golgi matrix components. These events are important for the breakdown of the nuclear envelope. At a later step, several kinesin-related motor proteins and cytoplasmic dynein are required for centrosome separation, mitotic spindle assembly, chromosome condensation, and Golgi fragmentation, respectively *(47,48)*. Furthermore,

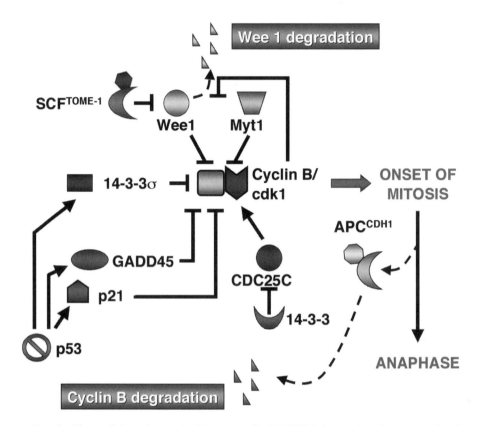

Fig. 3. The activity of mitotic kinase cyclin B/CDK1 is regulated at many levels before and during mitosis. Cyclin B/CDK1 is essential for the onset of mitosis. Inhibitory phosphorylation of Tyr15 (by Wee1) and Thr 14 and Tyr 15 (by Myt1) prevent the activation of CDK1. Protein phosphatase CDC25C removes inhibitory phosphoryl groups, allowing CDK1 activation. Before mitosis, CDC25C is sequestered in the cytoplasm by 14-3-3, whereas Wee1 is nuclear (Myt1 is cytoplasmic). At the onset of mitosis, the SCF complex targeted by Tome-1 degrades Wee1, thus tipping the balance in favor of CDK1 dephosphorylation. Once activated, cyclin B/CDK1 inactivates its own inhibitors, thus ensuring a positive feedback that leads to an abrupt increase in its activity and to the onset of mitosis. Before anaphase, the APC complex targeted by CDH1 degrades cyclin B, leading to loss of CDK1 activity and exit from mitosis. Under DNA damage conditions, the onset of mitosis is delayed by p53-dependent and -independent mechanisms (*see* **Subheading 4.**). In this example, active p53 prevents cyclin B/CDK1 activation via p21cip1/waf1, GADD45 and 14-3-3Σ. The latter sequesters cyclin B/CDK1 into the cytoplasm, preventing its nuclear activation. Other DNA damage-induced mechanisms include activation of Chk2 and Chk1 by DNA damage sensor ATM. These in turn phosphorylate CDC25C, favoring its cytoplasmic sequestration by 14-3-3. Pointed arrows indicate stimulation, whereas flat-tipped arrows indicate inhibition.

cyclin–B/CDK1 complexes contribute to regulate the anaphase-promoting complex/cyclosome (APC/C), the core component of the ubiquitin-dependent proteolytic machinery that controls the timely degradation of critical mitotic regulators *(47,48)*. In late telophase, cyclin B is ubiquitinated and degraded by the APC. This results in loss of CDK1 activity, exit from mitosis, and re-entry into interphase. APC in turn can be present in a complex with either CDC20 or CDH1. In yeast, CDC20-activated APC is involved in degradation of securin, which in turn inhibits the enzyme separase that is responsible for chromosome separation via degradation of cohesin *(47)*. Thus, CDC20-activated APC contributes to allowing chromosome separation. Conversely, CDH1-activated APC degrades cyclin B, resulting in exit from mitosis *(49)*. The subcellular localization of cyclin B/CDK1 effectors is crucial for the timing of kinase activation. The CDK1-inactivating kinase Wee1 is predominantly nuclear, whereas Myt1 is cytoplasmic. The CDC25C phosphatase is cytosolic until the G2/M transition, whereupon it is imported into the nucleus *(45,46,49)*. At the G2/M transition, Wee1 is degraded by the SCF complex. This complex targets different proteins for proteasome-mediated degradation depending on the F box subunit it contains *(49)*. Recently, an F-box protein that triggers Wee1 degradation has been identified and named "Tome-1" (Trigger of Mitotic Entry-1). In *Xenopus*, Tome-1 (which is conserved across species, including humans) interacts with Skp1 and CDC53 (otherwise known as Cul-1), forming an SCF complex that is required for Wee1 degradation and therefore for entry into mitosis *(49,50)*. The balance of activating and inhibitory influences on cyclin B/CDK1 controls the "switch" regulating entry into mitosis. This switch is controlled by MAP kinases, cell fate signals of many kinds, and by the DNA damage checkpoint *(19,45,47)*. Damage to DNA or the presence of unreplicated DNA prevents cyclin B/CDK1 activation by both p53-dependent and p53-independent mechanisms (**Fig. 2**). Through activation of ATM kinase and its downstream effectors chk1 and chk2, DNA damage triggers phosphorylation of CDC25C, which is then exported to the cytoplasm where it is retained as a complex with 14-3-3 protein. DNA damage also causes p53 activation through phosphorylation and acetylation. ATM is one of the factors that activate p53. Once active, p53 induces the expression of p21cip1/waf1, which is capable of inhibiting not just CDK2 but also CDK1, as well as other proteins that trigger G2 arrest, such as GADD45 and 14-3-3Σ. The latter sequesters cyclin B/CDK1 into the cytoplasm as an inactive complex. As a result of these events, cyclin B/CDK1 is prevented from being activated and from triggering mitosis while the cell attempts to correct the damage *(19)*.

Recent work has uncovered a whole array of other mitotic kinases that cooperate with cyclin B/CDK1 to control the progress of mitosis *(47)*. These include the Polo-like kinases, which appear to be required among other things for centrosome maturation *(51,52)*, the NIMA (Never in Mitosis A) family, which appears to play a role in separation of joined duplicated centrosomes, allowing the migration of the centrosomes at the two poles of the cell *(53,54)*, and the Aurora A, B, and C family kinases *(55–57)*, which localize to the centrosome and mitotic spindle microtubules (Aurora A), to the kinetocore and spindle midzone (Aurora B), and to the centrosome (Aurora C). Aurora A and B kinases are frequently overexpressed in tumor cells *(47)*. Additionally, the mitotic checkpoint kinases related to Bub1 participate in the "spindle assembly checkpoint," a mechanism that prevents anaphase until all kinetocores are properly connected with the mitotic spindle, and the "mitotic exit network" kinases participate in signaling cytokinesis at the end of mitosis *(47)*.

5. Transcriptional Functions of Cyclins/CDK: Cyclins Meet Ribonucleic Acid (RNA) Polymerase

A fundamental role of cyclin/CDKs that is often overlooked pertains to the control of RNA polymerase II (pol II)-mediated mRNA transcription. Specialized cyclins play pivotal roles in transcriptional control. Transcription is preceded by the formation of a preinitiation complex at promoter sites, containing general transcription factors TFIID, A, B, F, and H, as well as the pol II multisubunit holoenzyme. This complex melts the DNA double helix and can initiate transcription, but is unable to elongate the nascent mRNA. Elongation requires the phosphorylation of the C-terminal domain of the largest pol II subunit by a complex containing cyclin H, CDK7, and MAT-1 *(5,58)*. This complex is the same as CAK, the CDK-activating kinase, which activates CDK4 upon cyclin association (*see* **Subheading 2.1.**). This complex is also responsible for the phosphorylation of promoter-associated nuclear receptors such as the estrogen receptor α (ERα) or retinoid receptor RAR *(5)*. Additional positive and negative regulatory factors control mRNA elongation. Among these, the positive elongation regulator P-TEFb consists of CDK9 in association with one of the following cyclins: T1, T2, or K *(5,59,60)*. Thus, the successful transcription of polII-dependent genes is strictly dependent upon at least two specialized cyclin/CDK complexes.

6. Conclusion: Cyclin/CDK Complexes as Therapeutic Targets

The vast majority of antineoplastic drugs currently available and under development interfere with the cell cycle either directly or indirectly. Cytostatic drugs slow or block cell proliferation, while cytotoxic drugs trigger cell death, often through the activation of cell stress, DNA damage, or mitotic checkpoints in cells that are unable to arrest their cell cycle. The cell cycle machinery is almost universally altered in transformed cells. The G1 checkpoint in particular is virtually always disabled through a variety of mechanisms such as loss of p16INK4A, loss or Rb, overexpression of cyclin D1 or overexpression of CDK4. Loss or mutation of p53, among its many effects, weakens both the G1 and DNA damage checkpoints. Thus, it is not surprising that cyclin/CDK complexes have been at the center of considerable interest as potential therapeutic targets *(19,61–63)*. Various strategies have been used to restore the G1 checkpoint, from genetic reintegration of CKIs (either p16 or the CIP/KIP CKIs) to small-molecule CDK inhibitors *(19)*. The first approach is potentially more specific, but suffers from the well-known targeting and delivery problems that still beset the field of gene therapy. The small-molecule approach is potentially more practical, but is not without its own problems. First-generation CDK inhibitors such as flavopiridol or UCN-01, which have been studied in the clinic, are neither specific for CDKs nor, especially flavopiridol, function only as kinase inhibitors. Although these compounds appear to be reasonably safe and well tolerated, they have only modest clinical activity as single agents, and their in vivo mechanism(s) of action are far from clear. However, it is possible that they may be clinically useful in combination regimens with other chemotherapeutic agents. More specific CDK inhibitors are being developed. Still, the majority of these compounds target kinases in their ATP-binding sites. These sites are generally highly conserved throughout evolution, and thus, generating truly target-specific drugs using this approach is likely to prove rather difficult. High target specificity may not even be desirable from a therapeutic standpoint, given the extensive functional redundancy among cyclin/CDKs in mammalian cells. Targeting the interaction surfaces between cyclins and their cognate CDKs may eventually produce useful therapeutic agents, but it involves more complex drug development approaches than the identification of ATP analogs. Proof of concept for this approach has been obtained. For example, short peptides that block the interaction between cyclin A and CDK2 cause S-phase arrest and apoptosis in a way that appears to be selective for transformed cells *(64)*. Another possible approach may involve targeting the contact surfaces between CDKs and their substrates. Structural specificity is built into these surfaces, and thus drugs that interfere with them may affect specific CDK-mediated post-translational modification.

As far as the G2 checkpoint is concerned, strategies that prevent the inactivation of cyclin B/CDK1, thereby bypassing the DNA damage checkpoint, have shown promise, especially in association with DNA-damaging drugs. Methylxanthines such as caffeine inhibit ATM, whereas UCN-01 inhibits chk1 *(19)*. In both cases, the result in vitro is an increase in radiosensitivity due to partial disabling of the DNA damage checkpoint. Unfortunately, the doses of methylxanthines required for this effect are toxic in vivo, and UCN-01 has limited specificity. However, if specific inhibitors of ATM, chk1 or chk2 can be identified, it is likely that they will have radiosensitizing effects, and may synergize with DNA damaging drugs such anthracyclines or platinum compounds. Direct inhibition of cyclin B/CDK1, which in principle should cause failure to enter mitosis or premature exit from mitosis, has received comparatively less attention, but is in principle a valid strategy *(65)*. Next-generation CDK1 inhibitors are currently being developed *(66)*. Molecular studies on the regulation of cyclin/CDKs have revealed a prominent role for regulated proteolysis. This is often triggered by specialized E3 ubiquitin ligases that target cell key cycle regulators such as cyclin D1, p53, Wee1, or cyclin B for degradation. Phosphorylation at specific sites often increases the affinity of molecules to be targeted for degradation for their cognate E3 ligases. This suggests that manipulation of regulated proteolysis may be a potential alternative point of attack for the development of anti-neoplastic agents *(61,67,68)*.

In conclusion, a massive effort on the part of thousands of research groups over two decades has elucidated many of the fundamental mechanisms of cell cycle and cell fate control by cyclin/CDK complexes and many functions of cyclin/CDKs beyond cell cycle control. Several lessons can be drawn from these studies. On the one hand, the cell cycle field has demonstrated the great usefulness of simple unicellular or invertebrate models to identify key, evolutionarily conserved mediators of fundamental cellular processes. On the other hand, we have learned that simply identifying a crucial mediator of a biological process does not necessarily mean that this mediator will be a useful therapeutic target in humans. There are several reasons for this. The first is the massive redundancy observed in complex organisms, the likely result of gene duplication events that occurred during evolution. With few, if any, exceptions, crucial mediators identified in simple organisms are replaced in mammalian cells by whole families of structurally related molecules, whose functions partially overlap. This offers ample opportunities for a malignancy to escape the effects of highly specific inhibitors of one particular kinase by simply utilizing a related kinase (e.g., by selecting cells that overexpress the "replacement" kinase). With the possible exception of mutant/chimeric kinases such as Bcr/Abl, the idea of identifying an individual enzyme that is indispensable to neoplastic cells but not to normal cells, and can thus be targeted by highly specific inhibitors without fear of resistance, appears to be simplistic in light of what we know today. The identification of compounds that are highly specific for a family of kinases and do not affect other families at therapeutically useful concentrations is a difficult, though not necessarily impossible task. The second challenge facing experimental therapeutic efforts targeting cyclin/CDKs in humans is the law of unexpected consequences. To put it simply, the more fundamentally important a molecule is in cell biology, the more likely it is that interfering with it in humans will have unexpected effects on organs and systems other than the disease targets. This is owing to the fact that cyclin/CDKs, like other crucial mediators of cell fate, have been reused again and again during evolution for multiple functions. Thus, the idea that inhibiting a single kinase will block just a single or a handful of biological processes is generally unrealistic. What this means in practice is that there is no foolproof substitute for pilot clinical studies in the development of novel therapeutic agents. For example, a subtle neurological side effect that could grossly impair humans but is not necessarily evident in animal models would likely go undetected in pre-clinical studies. Knockout animals can provide some guidance in this respect, keeping in mind that these models are highly specific for the single gene being inactivated. Thus, they may or may not provide information that can be extrapolated to a drug that affects multiple targets in vivo.

All this does not necessarily mean that efforts aimed at developing therapeutically useful agents that interfere with cyclin/CDKs are doomed to failure. However, it does mean that future efforts will have to be more sophisticated than classical kinase inhibitor drug discovery efforts. Targeting the regulatory molecules that control cyclin/CDKs, targeting the interaction between CDKs and their substrates, inhibiting structurally related classes of kinases rather than single enzymes, attacking CDK-based signaling networks that are altered in cancer cells at multiple sites simultaneously, or using CDK inhibitors in timed combinations with agents that are likely to synergize with them are all potentially viable strategies. There is little doubt that once more sophisticated tools are developed to manipulate the activity of cyclin/CDKs, successful therapeutic applications will be within our grasp.

Acknowledgments

The author is supported by NIH (CA85064) and the Department of Defense Congressionally Directed Breast Cancer Initiative.

References

1. Evans, T., Rosenthal, E. T., Youngblom, J., Distel, D., and Hunt, T. (1983) Cyclin: a protein specified by maternal mRNA in sea urchin eggs that is destroyed at each cleavage division. *Cell* **33,** 389–396.
2. Blagosklonny, M. V. and Pardee, A. B. (2002) The restriction point of the cell cycle. *Cell Cycle* **1,** 103–110.
3. Sherr, C. J. (1995). D-type cyclins. *Trends Biochem. Sci.* **20,** 187–190.
4. Hunter, T. and Pines, J. (1994) Cyclins and cancer II: Cyclin D and CDK inhibitors come of age. *Cell* **79,** 573–582.
5. Coqueret, O. (2002) Linking cyclins to transcriptional control. *Gene* **299,** 35–55.
6. Morgan, D. O. (1997) Cyclin-dependent kinases: engines, clocks, and microprocessors. *Annu. Rev. Cell Dev. Biol.* **13,** 261–291.
7. Morgan, D. O. (1995) Principles of CDK regulation. *Nature* **374,** 131–134.

8. Russell, P. and Nurse, P. (1987) Negative regulation of mitosis by wee1+, a gene encoding a protein kinase homolog. *Cell* **49,** 559–567.

9. Russell, P. and Nurse, P. (1986) cdc25+ functions as an inducer in the mitotic control of fission yeast. *Cell* **45,** 145–153.

10. Harbour, J. W. and Dean, D. C. (2000) Chromatin remodeling and Rb activity. *Curr. Opin. Cell Biol.* **12,** 685–689.

11. Harbour, J. W. and Dean, D. C. (2001) Corepressors and retinoblastoma protein function. *Curr. Top. Microbiol. Immunol.* **254,** 137–144.

12. Harbour, J. W., Luo, R. X., Dei, S. A., Postigo, A. A., and Dean, D. C. (1999) Cdk phosphorylation triggers sequential intramolecular interactions that progressively block Rb functions as cells move through G1. *Cell* **98,** 859–869.

13. Harbour, J. W. and Dean, D. C. (2000) Rb function in cell-cycle regulation and apoptosis. *Nat. Cell Biol.* **2,** E65-E67.

14. Harbour, J. W. and Dean, D. C. (2000) The Rb/E2F pathway: expanding roles and emerging paradigms. *Genes Dev.* **14,** 2393–2409.

15. Sherr, C. J. (2000) The Pezcoller lecture: cancer cell cycles revisited. *Cancer Res.* **60,** 3689–3695.

16. Sherr, C. J. and Roberts, J. M. (1999) CDK inhibitors: positive and negative regulators of G1-phase progression. *Genes Dev.* **13,** 1501–1512.

17. Enders, G. H. (2003) The INK4a/ARF locus and human cancer. *Methods Mol. Biol.* **222,** 197–209.

18. Ortega, S., Malumbres, M., and Barbacid, M. (2002) Cyclin D-dependent kinases, INK4 inhibitors and cancer. *Biochim. Biophys. Acta* **1602,** 73–87.

19. Shapiro, G. I. and Harper, J. W. (1999) Anticancer drug targets: cell cycle and checkpoint control. *J. Clin. Invest.* **104,** 1645–1653.

20. Lowe, S. W. and Sherr, C. J. (2003) Tumor suppression by Ink4a-Arf: progress and puzzles. *Curr. Opin. Genet. Dev.* **13,** 77–83.

21. Sherr, C. J. and McCormick, F. (2002) The RB and p53 pathways in cancer. *Cancer Cell* **2,** 103–112.

22. Tetsu, O. and McCormick, F. (2003) Proliferation of cancer cells despite CDK2 inhibition. *Cancer Cell* **3,** 233–245.

23. Nickoloff, B. J., Osborne, B. A., and Miele, L. (2003) Notch signaling as a therapeutic target in cancer: a new approach to the development of cell fate modifying agents. *Oncogene* **22,** 6598–6608.

24. Yu, Z. K., Gervais, J. L., and Zhang, H. (1998) Human CUL-1 associates with the SKP1/SKP2 complex and regulates p21(CIP1/WAF1) and cyclin D proteins. *Proc. Natl. Acad. Sci. USA* **95,** 11,324–11,329.

25. Diehl, J. A., Cheng, M., Roussel, M. F., and Sherr, C. J. (1998) Glycogen synthase kinase-3beta regulates cyclin D1 proteolysis and subcellular localization. *Genes Dev.* **12,** 3499–3511.

26. Diehl, J. A., Zindy, F., and Sherr, C. J. (1997) Inhibition of cyclin D1 phosphorylation on threonine-286 prevents its rapid degradation via the ubiquitin-proteasome pathway. *Genes Dev.* **11,** 957–972.

27. Lustig, B. and Behrens, J. (2003) The Wnt signaling pathway and its role in tumor development. *J. Cancer Res. Clin. Oncol.* **129,** 199–221.

28. Manoukian, A. S. and Woodgett, J. R. (2002) Role of glycogen synthase kinase-3 in cancer: regulation by Wnts and other signaling pathways. *Adv. Cancer Res.* **84,** 203–229.

29. Raught, B., Gingras, A. C., and Sonenberg, N. (2001) The target of rapamycin (TOR) proteins. *Proc. Natl. Acad. Sci. USA* **98,** 7037–7044.

30. Schmelzle, T. and Hall, M. N. (2000) TOR, a central controller of cell growth. *Cell* **103,** 253–262.

31. Thomas, G. and Hall, M. N. (1997) TOR signalling and control of cell growth. *Curr. Opin. Cell Biol.* **9,** 782–787.

32. Duman-Scheel, M., Weng, L., Xin, S., and Du, W. (2002) Hedgehog regulates cell growth and proliferation by inducing cyclin D and cyclin E. *Nature* **417,** 299–304.

33. Shoker, B. S., Jarvis, C., Davies, M. P., Iqbal, M., Sibson, D. R., and Sloane, J. P. (2001) Immunodetectable cyclin D(1)is associated with oestrogen receptor but not Ki67 in normal, cancerous and precancerous breast lesions. *Br. J. Cancer* **84,** 1064–1069.

34. Zwijsen, R. M., Buckle, R. S., Hijmans, E. M., Loomans, C. J., and Bernards, R. (1998) Ligand-independent recruitment of steroid receptor coactivators to estrogen receptor by cyclin D1. *Genes Dev.* **12,** 3488–3498.

35. McMahon, C., Suthiphongchai, T., DiRenzo, J., and Ewen, M. E. (1999) P/CAF associates with cyclin D1 and potentiates its activation of the estrogen receptor. *Proc. Natl. Acad. Sci. USA* **96,** 5382–5387.

36. Lin, H. M., Zhao, L., and Cheng, S. Y. (2002) Cyclin D1 is a ligand-inde-pendent co-repressor for thyroid hormone receptors. *J. Biol. Chem.* **277,** 28,733–28,741.

37. Adnane, J., Shao, Z., and Robbins, P. D. (1999) Cyclin D1 associates with the TBP-associated factor TAF(II)250 to regulate Sp1-mediated transcription. *Oncogene* **18,** 239–247.

38. Sicinski, P. and Weinberg, R. A. (1997) A specific role for cyclin D1 in mammary gland development. *J. Mammary Gland. Biol. Neoplasia.* **2,** 335–342.

39. Sicinski, P., Donaher, J. L., Parker, S. B., Li, T., Fazeli, A., Gardner, H., et al. (1995) Cyclin D1 provides a link between development and oncogenesis in the reti-na and breast. *Cell* **82,** 621–630.

40. Geng, Y., Whoriskey, W., Park, M. Y., Bronson, R. T., Medema, R. H., Li, T., Weinberg, R. A., et al. (1999) Rescue of cyclin D1 deficiency by knockin cyclin E. *Cell* **97,** 767–777.

41. Ye, X., Wei, Y., Nalepa, G., and Harper, J. W. (2003) The cyclin E/Cdk2 substrate p220(NPAT) is required for S-phase entry, histone gene expression, and cajal body maintenance in human somatic cells. *Mol. Cell Biol.* **23,** 8586–8600.

42. Zhao, J., Kennedy, B. K., Lawrence, B. D., Barbie, D. A., Matera, A. G., Fletcher, J. A., et al. (2000) NPAT links cyclin E-Cdk2 to the regulation of replication-dependent histone gene transcription. *Genes Dev.* **14,** 2283–2297.

43. Yam, C. H., Fung, T. K., and Poon, R. Y. (2002) Cyclin A in cell cycle control and cancer. *Cell Mol. Life Sci.* **59,** 1317–1326.

44. Nevins, J. R., Chellappan, S. P., Mudryj, M., Hiebert, S., Devoto, S., Horowitz, J., et al. (1991) E2F transcription factor is a target for the RB protein and the cyclin A protein. *Cold Spring Harb. Symp. Quant. Biol.* **56,** 157–162.

45. O'Farrell, P. H. (2001) Triggering the all-or-nothing switch into mitosis. *Trends Cell Biol.* **11,** 512–519.

46. Mueller, P. R., Coleman, T. R., Kumagai, A., and Dunphy, W. G. (1995) Myt1: a membrane-associated inhibitory kinase that phosphorylates cdc2 on both threonine-14 and tyrosine-15. *Science* **270,** 86–90.

47. Nigg, E. A. (2001) Mitotic kinases as regulators of cell division and its checkpoints. *Nat. Rev. Mol. Cell Biol.* **2,** 21–32.

48. Nigg, E. A. (2001) Cell cycle regulation by protein kinases and phosphatases. *Ernst. Schering. Res. Found. Workshop* 19–46.

49. Lim, H. H. and Surana, U. (2003) Tome-1, wee1, and the onset of mitosis: coupled destruction for timely entry. *Mol. Cell* **11,** 845–846.

50. Ayad, N. G., Rankin, S., Murakami, M., Jebanathirajah, J., Gygi S., and Kirschner, M. W. (2003) Tome-1, a trigger of mitotic entry, is degraded during G1 via the APC. *Cell* **113,** 101–113.

51. Dai, W., Huang, X., and Ruan, Q. (2003) Polo-like kinases in cell cycle checkpoint control. *Front Biosci.* **8,** d1128–d1133.

52. Dai, W., Wang, Q., and Traganos, F. (2002) Polo-like kinases and centrosome regulation. *Oncogene* **21,** 6195–6200.

53. Fry, A. M. (2002) The Nek2 protein kinase: a novel regulator of centrosome structure. *Oncogene* **21,** 6184–6194.

54. Ye, X. S. and Osmani, S. A. (1997) Regulation of p34cdc2/cyclinB H1 and NIMA kinases during the G2/M transition and checkpoint responses in Aspergillus nidulans. *Prog. Cell Cycle Res.* **3,** 221–232.

55. Ke, Y. W., Dou, Z., Zhang, J., and Yao, X. B. (2003) Function and regulation of Aurora/Ipl1p kinase family in cell division. *Cell Res.* **13,** 69–81.

56. Adams, R. R., Carmena, M., and Earnshaw, W. C. (2001) Chromosomal passengers and the (aurora) ABCs of mitosis. *Trends Cell Biol.* **11,** 49–54.

57. Goepfert, T. M. and Brinkley, B. R. (2000) The centrosome-associated aurora/Ipl-like kinase family. *Curr. Top. Dev. Biol.* **49,** 331–342.

58. Shiekhattar, R., Mermelstein, F., Fisher, R. P., Drapkin, R., Dynlacht, B., Wessling, H. C., et al. (1995) Cdk-activating kinase complex is a component of human transcription factor TFIIH. *Nature* **374,** 283–287.

59. Lin, X., Taube, R., Fujinaga, K., and Peterlin, B. M. (2002) P-TEFb containing cyclin K and Cdk9 can activate transcription via RNA. *J. Biol. Chem.* **277,** 16,873–16,878.

60. Taube, R., Lin, X., Irwin, D., Fujinaga, K., and Peterlin, B. M. (2002) Interaction between P-TEFb and the C-terminal domain of RNA polymerase II activates transcriptional elongation from sites upstream or downstream of target genes. *Mol. Cell Biol.* **22,** 321–331.

61. Buolamwini, J. K. (2000) Cell cycle molecular targets in novel anticancer drug discovery. *Curr. Pharm. Des.* **6,** 379–392.

62. Senderowicz, A. M. (2003) Small-molecule cyclin-dependent kinase modulators. *Oncogene* **22,** 6609–6620.
63. Fischer, P. M. (2001) Recent advances and new directions in the discovery and development of cyclin-dependent kinase inhibitors. *Curr. Opin. Drug Dis. Dev.* **4,** 623–634.
64. Chen, Y. N., Sharma, S. K., Ramsey, T. M., Jiang, L., Martin, M. S., Baker, K., et al. (1999) Selective killing of transformed cells by cyclin/cyclin-dependent kinase 2 antagonists. *Proc. Natl. Acad. Sci. USA* **96,** 4325–4329.
65. Castedo, M., Perfettini, J. L., Roumier, T., and Kroemer, G. (2002) Cyclin-dependent kinase-1: linking apoptosis to cell cycle and mitotic catastrophe. *Cell Death Differ.* **9,** 1287–1293.
66. Seong, Y. S., Min, C., Li, L., Yang, J. Y., Kim, S. Y., Cao, X., et al. (2003) Characterization of a novel cyclin-dependent kinase 1 inhibitor, BMI-1026. *Cancer Res.* **63,** 7384–7391.
67. Dragnev, K. H., Freemantle, S. J., Spinella, M. J., and Dmitrovsky, E. (2001) Cyclin proteolysis as a retinoid cancer prevention mechanism. *Ann. N.Y. Acad. Sci.* **952,** 13–22.
68. Rolfe, M., Chiu, M. I., and Pagano, M. (1997) The ubiquitin-mediated proteolytic pathway as a therapeutic area. *J. Mol. Med.* **75,** 5–17.

2

In Situ Immunofluorescence Analysis

Immunofluorescence Microscopy

Amjad Javed, Sayyed K. Zaidi, Soraya E. Gutierrez,
Christopher J. Lengner, Kimberly S. Harrington, Hayk Hovhannisyan,
Brian C. Cho, Jitesh Pratap, Shirwin M. Pockwinse, Martin Montecino,
André J. van Wijnen, Jane B. Lian, Janet L. Stein, and Gary S. Stein

1. Introduction

Immunofluorescence is one of the most widely used techniques to study the localization of transcription factors, proteins, and structural components of nuclear architecture and cytoarchitecture. High-resolution *in situ* immunofluorescence approaches permit assessment of functional interrelationships between nuclear structure and gene expression that are linked to the intranuclear compartmentalization of nucleic acids and regulatory proteins (an example is shown in **Fig. 1**). The success of this method is dependent on the quality and specificity of the antibodies and the relative stability of antigens. Generally, the overall scheme for localization of cellular proteins involves fixation and permeabilization of cells for antibody accessibility, blocking, and staining with specific antibodies before microscopic examination. To reveal the subcellular and subnuclear macromolecular complexes that comprise and govern activation of the regulatory machinery for gene expression, cells can be subjected to selective extractions before immunodetection as described below.

2. Materials

1. Sterile glass cover slips (Fisher) coated with 0.5% gelatin (Life Technologies).
2. Cytoskeleton (CSK) buffer: (10× stock solution): 1 M NaCl, 100 mM PIPES, pH 6.8, 30 mM MgCl$_2$, 10 mM ethylenebis (oxyethylenenitrilo) tetraacetic acid (EGTA), 5% Triton X-100. (1× working solution): Freshly prepare 100 mL of 1× CSK buffer by dissolving 10.27 g sucrose in 77.6 mL of double-distilled water.

From: *Methods in Molecular Biology, Vol. 285: Cell Cycle Control and Dysregulation Protocols*
Edited by: A. Giordano and G. Romano © Humana Press Inc., Totowa, NJ

RUNX2 DAPI DIC

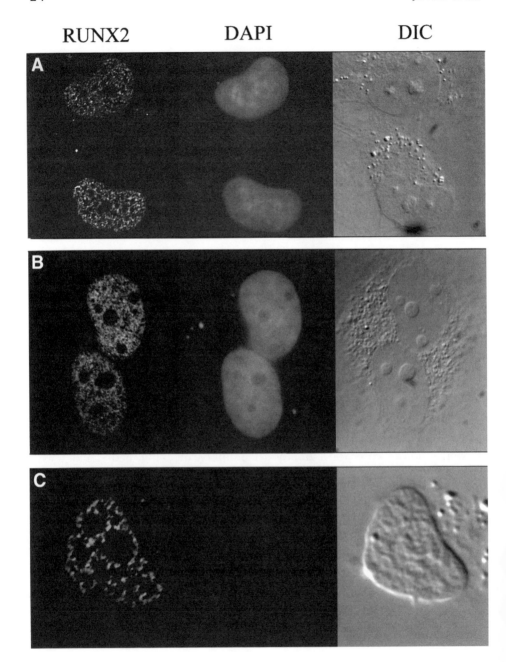

Fig. 1. *In situ* immunofluorescence detection of transcription factors at intranuclear sites. Runx/Cbfa/AML transcription factors provide an example of regulatory proteins that can be detected *in situ*. HeLa cells grown on gelatin-coated cover slips were transiently transfected with 0.5 μg of Runx2 expression plasmid, using "SuperFect" reagent (Qiagen Inc, CA). Cells were processed 20 h later for *in situ* detection of Run μ2 in intact cells (**A**) or after removal of cytoskeletal component (**B**) or in nuclear matrix preparations (**C**). Run μ2 proteins were detected with a rabbit polyclonal Run μ2 antibody and an fluorescein isothiocyanate-conjugated antirabbit secondary antibody. DAPI detects deoxyribonucleic acid (DNA) in nuclei of whole cells and CSK extracted cells but not in NMIF preparations because DNA has been digested and extracted. Differential interference contrast microscopy shows a bright field image of cells. The punctate, non-nucleolar distribution of Run μ2 protein is preserved throughout the extraction procedure. Original magnification × 63.

Add 10 mL of 10× stock CSK buffer, (Sigma), 0.8 mL of ribonucleoside–vanadyl complex (RVC) (New England Biolabs) and 0.2 mL of 400 mM 4-[2-aminoethyl] benzenesulfonyl fluoride (AEBSF).

3. Digestion buffer (DB): (10× Stock Solution): 0.5 M NaCl, 100 mM PIPES, pH 6.8, 30 mM MgCl$_2$, 10 mM EGTA 5% Triton X-100. Freshly prepare 1× DB as described above for 1× CSK buffer except for using 10× DB instead of 10× CSK buffer.

4. Phosphate-buffered saline (PBS): 9.1 mM dibasic sodium phosphate, 1.7 mM monobasic sodium phosphate, and 150 mM NaCl. Adjust pH to 7.4 with NaOH.

5. Fixatives: 3.7% formaldehyde in PBS (WC fixative), or in 1× CSK buffer (CSK fixative), or in 1× DB (nuclear matrin intermediate filament [NMIF] fixative). All fixatives should be freshly prepared.

6. Stop solution: 250 mM ammonium sulfate in 1× DB. (Add 1 volume of 2 M ammonium sulfate to 8 volume of 1× DB).

7. Permeabilizing solution: 0.25% Triton X-100 in PBS.

8. PBSA: 0.5% bovine serum albumin (BSA) in PBS. **Note:** Filter sterilize all solutions before use.

3. Methods
3.1. Whole Cell (WC) Preparation

Note: This method is for adherent cells. Biochemical sub cellular fractionation can be performed as described in **Fig. 2.**

1. Plate cells at a density of 0.5×10^6 cells per well and incubate in humidified incubator at 37°C.

2. After 24 h, wash cells twice with ice-cold PBS.

Biochemical Fractionation

Two 100mm plates per construct

Scrape cells in 1ml of 1XPBS containing
protease inhibitor cocktail

Harvest cells in 300µl of direct
lysis buffer; collect cell slurry,
boil for 5 min. (**"WC" fraction**)

↓

Collect cells by centrifugation
at 14,000rpm for 15 seconds

↓

Extract cell pellet with 150µl of CSK buffer for 10 minutes on ice

↓

Spin samples at 14,000rpm for 10 minutes and transfer
the supernatant to a clean tube (**"CSK fraction"**)

↓

Repeat CSK extraction as above, pool the supernatant with previous one

↓

Resuspend pellet in 150µl Digestion buffer containing
400U/ml of DNaseI for 25 minutes at room temperature

↓

Spin samples at 14,000rpm for 10 minutes, collect
supernatant (**"Nuclease fraction"**)

↓

Repeat extraction with Digestion buffer as above, add ammonium sulfate to
obtain a final concentration of 250mM, extract for additional 5 minutes

↓

Spin for 10 min. at 14,000rpm, collect and
pool supernatant with nuclease fraction

↓

Resuspend pellet in 300µl of Direct lysis
buffer; boil for 5 minutes (**"NM-IF"**)

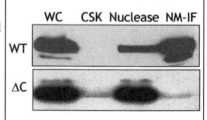

Fig. 2. Protocol overview for biochemical detection of regulatory molecules in subcellular compartments. A stepwise schematic diagram indicates the procedures required for detection of regulatory proteins in subcellular and subnuclear components of cell by biochemical fractionation. HeLa cells were transiently transfected with HA-tagged RUNμ2 expression constructs for wild type (1-528 amino-acids) and C-terminal deletion mutant ΔC (1-376 amino-acids). Cell pellets were subjected to extraction buffers and different fractions were collected as indicated. Equal volumes (30 μL) of all fractions were separated on a 10% sodium dodecyl sulfate polyacrylamide gel electrophoresis. The proteins were immobilized onto a polyvinylidene difluoride membrane (Millipore) and probed with monoclonal anti-HA antibody. The full-length protein (WT) is resistant to high salt extraction and is tightly bound with the nuclear matrix. However the mutant protein (ΔC) is not associated with the nuclear matrix and is released into the nuclease fraction.

3. Fix the WC preparation on ice for 10 min (typically two wells of a six-well plate) by adding 2 mL of WC fixative per well.
4. Wash cells once with PBS.
5. To facilitate antibody staining of WC preparations, permeabilize WC preparations with 1 mL of permeabilizing solution on ice for 20 min.
6. Aspirate permeabilizing solution and wash twice with PBS.
7. Add 1 mL of PBSA in the wells.

3.2. Cytoskeleton (CSK) Preparation

If further subcellular fractionation is required, we recommend extraction be performed first followed by fixation and antibody labeling as described below.

1. Wash cells twice with ice-cold PBS.
2. Add 1 mL of 1× CSK buffer per well and incubate plates on ice for 15 min while swirling plates every 2–3 min.
3. Aspirate CSK buffer and add fresh 1 mL of 1× CSK buffer and incubate plates on ice for additional 15 min while swirling plates every 2–3 min.
4. Wash wells for CSK preparation (typically two wells of six well plates) once with ice-cold PBS and fix cells by adding 2 mL of CSK fixative per well.
5. Aspirate CSK fixative after 10 min and wash twice with PBS.
6. Add 1 mL of PBSA to the wells.

3.3. NMIF Preparation

1. Follow **steps 1–3** of **Subheading 3.1.2.**
2. Wash cells once with ice-cold PBS.
3. Prepare 1 mL of DB by adding 400 U of RNase free DNase I (Roche) to 1× DB.

4. Flattened parafilm on the covers of plates and dispense 20 µL drop of DB containing RNase free DNase I on the covers of respective plates. (This step is to conserve the amount of DNase I; otherwise, add 1 mL of DB containing RNase free DNase I to each well.)

5. Carefully place the cover slips for digestion of the chromatin with DNase I so that cells will face DB containing DNase I.

6. Incubate cells for 20 min at room temperature (20–22°C). In case the digestion with DNase I is partial (different degrees of low intensity signals will be detected with DAPI stain), we recommend carrying out first digestion at 28°C and second at room temperature. Place cover slips back in their respective wells, wipe the DB from the covers and repeat the DNase I digestion.

7. Place cover slips back in their respective wells. Add 1mL stop solution to the wells and incubate plates on ice for 10 min to stop the activity of DNase I.

8. Wash once with ice-cold PBS and fix NMIF preparations in 2 mL of NMIF fixative on ice for 10 min.

9. Aspirate fixative and wash twice with PBS.

10. Add 1 mL of PBSA.

3.4. Immunostaining of the Samples

1. Dilute antibody in PBSA to an appropriate dilution. We recommend several dilutions to be tested as quality and specificity of antibodies vary among suppliers and lots. While immunolabeling cells for two proteins, caution must be practiced to assure that the antibodies used are raised in different species (e.g., mouse vs rabbit). If raised in same species, they must be of different isotypes (e.g., IgG vs IgM).

2. Dispense a 20-µL drop of antibody dilution for each well on parafilm already flattened on the lids of plates. Carefully place cover slip on the drop so that the cells are in direct contact with the antibody. Avoid creating air bubble by gently placing the cover slips from one edge on the antibody. Incubate for 1 h at 37°C.

3. Place cover slips back in respective wells with cells facing upward and wash four times with ice-cold PBSA.

4. Stain cells with appropriate secondary antibodies conjugated with fluorochromes (e.g., Texas Red or fluorescein isothiocyanate) for 1 h at 37°C.

5. Place cover slips back in their respective wells and wash four times with ice-cold PBSA.

6. Stain cells with DAPI (0.5 µg of DAPI in 0.1% Triton × 100-PBSA) for 5 min on ice.

7. Wash once with 0.1% Triton × 100-PBSA followed by two washes with PBS. Leave cells in last wash on ice to avoid descication.

8. Immediately mount cover slips in antifade mounting medium (e.g., VectaShield) and air dry excess of mounting medium for 10–15 min. Seal cover slips and store at –20°C in the dark.

3

In Situ Immunofluorescence Analysis

Analyzing RNA Synthesis by 5-Bromouridine-5'-Triphosphate Labeling

Amjad Javed, Sayyed K. Zaidi, Soraya E. Gutierrez, Christopher J. Lengner, Kimberly S. Harrington, Hayk Hovhannisyan, Brian C. Cho, Jitesh Pratap, Shirwin M. Pockwinse, Martin Montecino, André J. van Wijnen, Jane B. Lian, Janet L. Stein, and Gary S. Stein

1. Introduction

This technique is used to visualize sites of active transcription in a permeabilized cell and does not require radiolabeled molecules (e.g., [^{3}H] Uridine). Nonradioactive ribonucleic acid (RNA) precursors (e.g., 5-bromouridine-5'-triphosphate [BrUTP]) are used and can be detected by using fluorescently labeled antibodies. Procedures for BrUTP of labeling transcription sites require manipulations that are best applied to adherent cells but can be applied, with difficulty, to cell cultures in suspension. The protocol described below is for adherent cells grown on cover slips.

2. Materials

2.1. Analyzing RNA Synthesis by BrUTP Labeling (see Notes 1–3)

1. BrUTP, 14.9 mM. Dissolve 10 mg of powdered BrUTP in 1 mL of dH$_2$O and add 2 M Tris-HCl, pH 7.4, to bring to pH 7. Store in 100 µL aliquots at –20°C.
2. 100 mM NTPs (Roche); store aliquots at –20°C.
3. 10 mM S-adenosylmethionine. Dissolve 5 mg in 1 mL of dH$_2$O and store aliquots at –20°C.
4. Glycerol buffer: 20 mM Tris-HCl, pH 7.4, 5 mM MgCl$_2$, 0.5 mM ethylenebis(oxyethylenenitrilo)tetraacetic acid (EGTA), 25% glycerol. For 500 mL of glycerol buffer, add 1.2 g Tris-HCl (or 10 mL of 1 M Tris-HCl, pH 7.4), 0.5 g

From: *Methods in Molecular Biology, Vol. 285: Cell Cycle Control and Dysregulation Protocols*
Edited by: A. Giordano and G. Romano © Humana Press Inc., Totowa, NJ

MgCl$_2$·6H$_2$O (or 2.5 mL of 1 M MgCl$_2$), 0.1 g EGTA (or 1 mL of 0.25 M EGTA), and 125 mL of 100% glycerol.

5. Glycerol buffer + 0.05% Triton X-100 + AEBSF: 20 mM Tris-HCl, pH 7.4, 5 mM MgCl$_2$, 0.5 mM EGTA, 25% glycerol, 0.05% Triton X-100, 1.6 mM AEBSF. For 2 mL of glycerol buffer + 0.05% Triton X-100 + AEBSF: 1.98 mL of glycerol buffer, 10 µL of 10% Triton X-100, and 8 µL of 400 mM AEBSF.

6. 2× Synthesis buffer: 100 mM Tris-HCl, pH 7.4, 20 mM MgCl$_2$·H$_2$O, 1 mM EGTA, 200 mM KCl, 50% glycerol. For 100 mL of 2× synthesis buffer: 1.2 g of Tris-HCl (or 10 mL of 1 M Tris-HCl, pH 7.4), 0.4g MgCl$_2$ (or 2 mL of 1 M MgCl$_2$), 0.04 g of EGTA (or 0.4 mL of 0.25 M EGTA), 1.5 g of KCl, and 50 mL of glycerol.

7. Transcription buffer: Freshly prepare 1 mL: 500 µL 2× synthesis buffer, 2.5 µL of 10 mM S-adenosylmethionine, 5 µL each 100 mM ATP, CTP, GTP, 50 µL 15 mM BrUTP, 4 µL 400 mM AEBSF, 1 µL RNase Inhibitor (Roche), and 420 µL of DEPC dH$_2$O.

3. Methods

3.1. Analyzing RNA Synthesis by BrUTP Labeling

1. Grow about 0.5 × 10^6 cells on gelatin coated cover slips for 24 h. Number of cells on the cover slip is important; as well spread cells (40–60% density) yield best results.
2. Wash cells with phosphate-buffered saline (PBS) twice.
3. Incubate 3 min in glycerol buffer.
4. Incubate 3 min in glycerol buffer + 0.05% Triton X-100 + AEBSF (we recommend titrating the minimum concentration of triton required to permeabilize the cells).
5. Incubate 15 min in transcription buffer (use at least 60 µL on each cover slip). Labeling time could be varied from 5 to 30 min.
6. Wash with PBS + AEBSF.
7. Cells may now be processed as usual for whole cell, cytoskeleton (CSK), or nuclear matrin intermediate filament (NMIF). (For details, see Chapter 2, **Subheading 3.1.1.**).

3.2. Cell Processing

3.2.1. Whole Cell Preparation

1. Fix cells for 10 min on ice in 3.7% formaldehyde in PBS.
2. Rinse cells twice with 1 mL of 1× PBS containing 2 mM ribonucleoside–vanadyl complex (RVC) and 1.6 mM AEBSF.
3. To facilitate antibody staining of WC preparations, permeabilize cells with 1mL of permeabilizing solution for 20 min.
4. Block with PBSA (0.5% BSA in PBS) containing 2 mM RVC and 1.6 mM AEBSF.

3.2.2. Cytoskeleton Preparation

1. Incubate on ice for 3 min in CSK buffer containing 0.5% Triton, RVC, and AEBSF.
2. Fix cells for 10 min on ice in CSK fixative (3.7% formaldehyde in CSK buffer).

3. Rinse with 1 mL of 1× PBS containing 2 m*M* RVC and 1.6 m*M* AEBSF.
4. Block with PBSA containing 2 m*M* RVC and 1.6 m*M* AEBSF.

3.2.3. Nuclear Matrix Intermediate Filament Preparation

1. Incubate cells on ice for 3 min in CSK buffer containing 0.5% Triton, RVC, and AEBSF.
2. Remove chromatin by incubating cells for 30 min at 30°C in 400U/mL DNase I (Roche) in DB containing 0.5% Triton, RVC, and AEBSF.
3. Extract cells with ammonium sulfate in DB containing 0.5% Triton, VRC, AEBSF for 10 min, and then for 1 min.
4. Fix cells for 10 min on ice with NMIF fixative (3.7% formaldehyde in DB buffer).
5. Rinse cells with 1 mL of 1× PBS containing 2m*M* RVC and 1.6 m*M* AEBSF.
6. Block cells with PBSA containing 2 m*M* RVC and 1.6 m*M* AEBSF.

3.3. Antibody Incubations

1. Primary antibodies are diluted in PBSA. Use 50 µL on each cover slip and cover with parafilm. Incubate for either 2 h at room temperature or at 4°C overnight. Antibodies to be used are Rat anti-BrdU, 1:25 Accurate Chemicals. This antibody and dilution have consistently yielded the best results in our laboratories when compared with other antibodies or different dilutions (*see ref. 1*); mouse anti-BrdU, 1:100 (Roche), and mouse anti-BrdU, 1:500 (Sigma).
2. Wash cells four times with PBSA.
3. Dilute secondary antibody goat-anti-rat Alena 488 or 594 in PBSA (1:800 dilution).
4. Use a 30 µl drop on each cover slip and cover with parafilm. Incubate cover slips at 37°C for 45 min.
5. Wash cells four times with PBSA.
6. Stain cells with DAPI for 4 min on ice in 1 mL of PBSA containing 0.5 µg DAPI and 1% Triton.
7. Wash cells once with PBSA containing 0.1% Triton.
8. Rinse cells twice with 1× PBS.
9. Mount cover slips in vectashield or ProLong (or other anti-fade mounting media).

4. Notes

1. For best results, use Roche RNase Inhibitor.
2. All solutions should be RNase-free.
3. Use DEPC-treated dH$_2$O to prepare solutions.

References

1. Wansink, D. G., Motley, A. M., van Driel, R., and de Jong, L. (1994) Fluorescent labeling of nascent RNA in the cell nucleus using 5-bromouridine 5′-triphosphate. in *Cell Biology—A Laboratory Handbook* (J. Celis, ed.), Academic Press, San Diego, CA, pp. 368–374.

4

Immunofluorescence Analysis Using Epitope-Tagged Proteins

In Vitro System

Amjad Javed, Sayyed K. Zaidi, Soraya E. Gutierrez, Christopher J. Lengner, Kimberly S. Harrington, Hayk Hovhannisyan, Brian C. Cho, Jitesh Pratap, Shirwin M. Pockwinse, Martin Montecino, André J. van Wijnen, Jane B. Lian, Janet L. Stein, and Gary S. Stein

1. Introduction

The resolution that can be attained in assessment of the intranuclear localization of cellular proteins is dependent on specificity of the antibodies. Primary antibodies should be well characterized. We recommend testing antibody specificity by immunoblotting. In general, monoclonal antibodies have a selective advantage of recognizing only a single epitope but may not produce a high titer. In contrast, polyclonal antibodies generally have a high titer but may recognize multiple epitopes that may result in crossreactivity with several proteins because of similar amino acid sequences. The problem of low titer antibody and poor antigenicity can be overcome by marking the proteins with an epitope "tag." The most widely used tags in prokaryotic and eukaryotic cells include glutathione S-transferase , β-galactosidase, 6× histidine, hemagglutinin, Xpress, Flag, Myc, and a variety of fluorescent proteins (green fluorescent protein [GFP], cyan fluorescent protein, yellow fluorescent protein, and red fluorescent protein). Caution must be exercised when tagging large proteins (e.g., GFP or β-galactosidase) at the amino or carboxy termini to avoid interference with folding that can influence activity. Most "epitope tags" are very short sequences, thereby having little or no crossreactivity with other cellular proteins. The well-characterized antibodies that are commercially available against these tags are also conjugated to fluorescent molecules. These

From: *Methods in Molecular Biology, Vol. 285: Cell Cycle Control and Dysregulation Protocols*
Edited by: A. Giordano and G. Romano © Humana Press Inc., Totowa, NJ

conjugated reagents reduce both the time and assessment of chemical needed to visualize the final product. Furthermore many vectors are now commercially available with signals to direct expressed proteins to specific sites and organelles in the cells.

Physiologic levels of proteins marked with different tags can be achieved by transfecting expression plasmids into cell types of choice. These cells can be processed to assess the functional distribution of the tagged molecule relative to endogenous protein. Caution must be exercised to prevent excessive expression of exogenous protein that can be targeted to subnuclear regions other than the native sites. The *in situ* assessment of tagged proteins can be conducted essentially following the protocol described in Chapters 2 and 3.

GFP is 238 amino acids long and was cloned in 1992. GFP is widely used as reporter molecule for monitoring gene expression and protein localization in vivo, *in situ*, and in real time. Detection of GFP does not require co-factors, enzyme substrates, or antibodies. Therefore, it can be followed in living cells, making it possible to study the dynamics of GFP-tagged proteins. Although originally cloned from the jellyfish *Aequorea victoria*, a humanized version (with silent mutations for human codon usage preference) designated EGFP, is available for maximal expression in mammalian cells. Because of the increase in its excitation coefficient, the EGFP is 35 times more intense than GFP.

The amount of plasmid deoxyribonucleic acid (DNA) required and the method of transfection vary depending on cell type. The quality of DNA is of prime importance. Lipid-based transfection reagents generally have low cytotoxicity and high transfection efficiency. We recommend pretesting the transfection conditions for optimal expression of GFP-tagged proteins.

2. Materials
2.1. Time-Lapse Imaging

1. Glass cover slips.
2. 0.5% Gelatin.
3. Mitotracker red CM-H2XRos dye (Molecular Probes, Eugene, OR). Reconstitute lyophilized Mitotracker dye in DMSO to a final concentration of 1 mM.
4. 1× PBS.
5. Phenol red free media: If the cell chamber is not equipped to use CO_2, change in pH of the media will occur. A constant pH can be maintained by using HEPES when making the media.
6. Transfection reagent.
7. FCS-2 closed cell chamber incubator (Bioptechs, Butler, PA).
8. Zeiss Axioplan 2 microscope with CCD camera.
9. Associated software and hardware for image storage and analysis.

3. Methods

3.1. Time-Lapse Imaging

1. Plate cells in 100-mm plates on 0.5% gelatin-coated 40-mm cover slips (Bioptechs, Butler, PA) at a density of 2×10^6 cells per plate and incubate in humidified incubator at 37°C.

2. Transfect cells with 2–4 μg of supercoiled expression plasmid DNA.

3. Incubate cells for 14–18 h in humidified incubator at 37°C after transfection. (We recommend preassessing the time frame required with your transfection conditions and cell type before performing the actual time lapse experiment.) The time by which a detectable amount of GFP-tagged protein is accumulated will depend on the promoter driving the GFP-tagged protein, the method of transfection, the cell type, and the transfection efficiency.

4. Dilute 1 mM Mitotracker red CM-H2XRos dye in a prewarmed complete medium (the medium in which cells are grown) to a final concentration of 100 nM to stain mitochondria. (The Mitotracker red dye is generally used as a marker for viability before and after capturing images since this dye is only fluorescent after oxidation by active mitochondria.)

5. Incubate cells for 30 min at 37°C.

6. Wash cells once with 5 mL of media and transfer cover slips to the cell chamber.

7. Remove cover slips from the 100-mm plate and assemble in the cell chamber with perfusing complete media without phenol red (Life Technologies) supplemented with 10 nM Mitotracker Red dye.

8. Set the FCS-2 closed cell chamber incubator (Bioptechs, Butler, PA) and objective heater to maintain cells at 37°C. Turn on other accessories after assembly of chamber (e.g., pump for continuous circulation of media during the course of time-lapse imaging) that are associated with the upright microscope.

9. Turn on the microscope for fluorescence imaging and locate the GFP-positive cell(s) to be followed. It is easier to locate the region of interest using low magnification and low intensity illumination.

10. Change to appropriate objective magnification before proceeding with actual recording. In general objective with high numerical aperture yields better results.

11. Cells vary in their sensitivity to radiation exposure. To reduce radiation damage, exposures can be obtained with low excitation intensity and increased signal accumulation time. Although short exposures under intense illumination yield crisp images with low background noise, it may cause more radiation damage to the cells. The exposure length and illumination intensity would also depend on the amount of GFP signal in the cell at the time of imaging.

12. Record images with an interval of 10–30 s for 20–30 min. Short intervals result in unnecessary photobleaching and cell damage and intervals that are too long may cause mistakes in interpretation of temporal changes or dynamic properties of the protein. If the protein in question is a signaling molecule and its dynamics is being studied in response to stimuli, the exposure interval may have to be much shorter.

12. The series of time-lapse images should be collected as an electronic stack file. Exposure times for GFP fusion protein range between 100 and 300 ms and for the Mitotracker Red dye between 100 and 500 ms. Different software are commercially available for automatic acquisition of images. When using longer periods for imaging, a drift in focus can occur because of cell movement or movement of microscope. It is difficult to eliminate the drift in the focus; however, stabilizing the temperature and capturing images for short periods of time at low magnification can reduce it.

13. The best and most effective way to analyze the series of data points is to play them as a movie. The series of images can be loaded into an image processor and differences are visualized by rapidly switching among these images, effectively creating a motion picture. Alternatively, the images can be displayed as a montage and changes in a selective area can be monitored.

5

Analysis of In Vivo Gene Expression Using Epitope-Tagged Proteins

Amjad Javed, Sayyed K. Zaidi, Soraya E. Gutierrez,
Christopher J. Lengner, Kimberly S. Harrington, Hayk Hovhannisyan,
Brian C. Cho, Jitesh Pratap, Shirwin M. Pockwinse, Martin Montecino,
André J. van Wijnen, Jane B. Lian, Janet L. Stein, and Gary S. Stein

1. Introduction

Only a handful of tagged molecules have been used successfully in vivo to monitor gene expression. The most commonly used are β-galactosidase (β-gal) and green fluorescent protein (GFP). Both molecules pose limitations with in vivo detection. When using GFP, autofluorescence may be encountered in tissues and tissue sections. Similarly, when using β-gal as a marker, the penetration of X-gal substrate is difficult in tissues with extensive extra cellular matrix and in calcified tissues

The *Escherichia coli* lacZ gene encoding β-gal is widely used as a reporter molecule for in vitro, in vivo, and transgenic applications. β-gal can be detected using a variety of substrates, all of which have galactose linked through a β-D-glycosidic linkage to a moiety whose properties change upon liberation from galactose. Several commercially available substrates yield colored or fluorescent soluble products that are useful when quantifying β-gal activity or visualizing transduced cells in vivo (an example is shown in **Fig. 1**). The procedure below is described for X-gal. When β-gal cleaves the glycosidic linkage in X-gal, a soluble, colorless indoxyl monomer is produced. Subsequently, two of the liberated indoxyl moieties form a dimer that is nonenzymatically oxidized. The resultant halogenated indigo is a very stable and insoluble blue compound. Alternative staining protocols that yield different colored products have been developed.

From: *Methods in Molecular Biology, Vol. 285: Cell Cycle Control and Dysregulation Protocols*
Edited by: A. Giordano and G. Romano © Humana Press Inc., Totowa, NJ

A   **B**

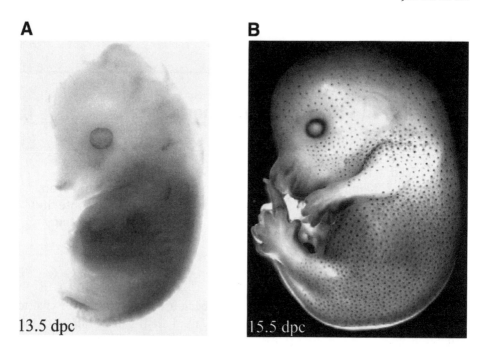

13.5 dpc   15.5 dpc

Fig. 1. Analysis of gene expression in vivo by a β-gal reporter. Whole-mount X-gal staining of transgenic embryos expressing the β-gal gene under the control of a mammalian promoter to indicate the transcriptional activity in vivo. Timed pregnant mothers of two different transgenic lines were sacrificed to harvest embryos at 13.5 dpc (**A**) or 15.5 dpc (**B**). The embryos were fixed overnight in paraformaldehyde–glutaraldehyde, rinsed in PBS, and left overnight in a solution containing X-gal, potassium ferricyanide and potassium ferrocyanide to detect β-gal activity. The soft tissues were clarified by placing 13.5 dpc embryos (**A**) in 2% KOH solution for 2 d. Stained embryos were then stored in solution containing 50% glycerol and 50% ethanol. Intense X-gal staining of the rib and vertebral column (**A**) and hair follicles (**B**) is evident.

2. Materials

1. 4% Paraformaldehyde.
2. 25% Glutaraldehyde.
3. 0.5 M Ethylenebis(oxyethylenenitrilo)tetraacetic acid (EGTA).
4. 1 M MgCl$_2$.
5. Rotating shaker.
6. Phosphate-buffered saline (PBS).
7. Potassium ferricyanide; store at 4°C.
8. Potassium ferrocyanide; store at 4°C.

9. Nonidet P-40.
10. 1% Sodium deoxycholate.
11. Dimethyl sulfoxide (DMSO).
12. X-gal stock (40 mg/mL) in DMSO.
13. X-gal reaction buffer (5 mM potassium ferrocyanide, 5 mM potassium ferricyanide, 2 mM MgCl$_2$, 0.02% NP-40, 0.01% sodium deoxycholate 1 mg/mL X-gal). The amount of potassium ferrocyanide and potassium ferricyanide used for staining may vary. To avoid X-gal precipitation, make fresh solution every time and store at 4°C in dark bottles.

3. Methods

1. Isolate mouse embryos from timed pregnant mother and remove to 1× PBS containing 2 mM MgCl$_2$.
2. Fix embryos in either fresh 4% paraformaldehyde (this is good for *in situ* hybridization), 10% phosphate-buffered formalin (when using histological sections), or a solution containing [2% paraformaldehyde, 0.2% glutaraldehyde, 5 mM EGTA, and 2 mM MgCl$_2$ in 1× PBS, pH 8.8].
3. Fixation times vary from 1 h [for 8.5- to 9.5-d post coitus (dpc) embryos] to overnight (for 15.5 dpc embryos) at 4°C. The time scale for fixation should be determined empirically. Generally, it is wise to minimize time in fixative, as the β-galactosidase can be overfixed. Older embryos may also be fixed but is not recommended because of poor infiltration. Larger embryos may be dissected and fixed in pieces. All fixations should be performed at 4°C with gentle shaking or rotating. It is important to use ample volume of fixative (50 mL per embryo from 13.5 to 15.5 dpc).
4. After fixation, rinse twice (30 min each) in 1× PBS. Alternatively rinse in many changes of PBS as residual fixative can inhibit the enzyme.
5. Stain tissues in X-gal reaction buffer containing 5 mM each of potassium ferricyanide and ferrocyanide, 2 mM MgCl$_2$, 0.2% NP40, 0.1% sodium deoxycholate, and 1 mg/mL X-gal made up in DMSO, all together in 1× PBS, pH 7.3. Staining times vary according to embryo size and temperature. Embryos that are 8.5–11.5 dpc can be stained at room temperature for about 6 h or at 37°C for about 2 h (*see* **Notes 1–4**).
6. Rinse in 1× PBS, pH 7.3, for a few hours after staining. We recommend rinsing many times in PBS until the solution no longer turns yellow. Tissues can then be stored at 4°C in 5% phosphate-buffered formalin or processed for sectioning in paraffin or other embedding medium.
7. View under bright-field optics for optimal detection.

4. Notes

1. Embryos (12.5–15.5 dpc) should be stained overnight at room temperature to ensure penetration.

2. All staining should be performed on shaking platform using ample volumes of stain (8.5–9.5 dpc, about 2 mL, 10.5–11.5 dpc, about 10 mL, 12.5–15.5 dpc, about 30 to 50 mL).

3. Older embryos 15.5 dpc+ do not exhibit reliable whole mount staining because of lack of penetration.

4. Tissues may be dissected and stained individually.

6

Chromatin Immunoprecipitation

Amjad Javed, Sayyed K. Zaidi, Soraya E. Gutierrez,
Christopher J. Lengner, Kimberly S. Harrington, Hayk Hovhannisyan,
Brian C. Cho, Jitesh Pratap, Shirwin M. Pockwinse, Martin Montecino,
André J. van Wijnen, Jane B. Lian, Janet L. Stein, and Gary S. Stein

1. Introduction

Fundamental parameters of biological control require sequence-specific protein–deoxyribonucleic acid (DNA) interactions. The packaging of DNA into higher order chromatin controls accessibility to DNA binding proteins that influence regulatory events that include transcription, replication, recombination, and DNA repair. Chromatin is remodeled in a physiologically responsive manner by covalently modifying histones to neutralize a positive charge of these basic chromosomal proteins that form nucleosomes, the primary unit of nucleoprotein structure. Acetylation and methylation of residues on the unstructured tails of histone proteins are the most prevalent chromatin modification related to transcriptional regulation. To understand chromatin structure of a gene, it is important to characterize the interactions of structural and regulatory proteins in the vicinity of covalently modified nucleosomes. Formaldehyde crosslinking rapidly fixes protein–protein and protein–DNA complexes in vivo providing the basis for an approach to analyze native structure of gene promoters. The protocol below is a simple yet sensitive method to determine whether a known protein is associated with a DNA sequence in mammalian cells. It must be noted that this protocol is not limited to sequence-specific DNA binding proteins. The success of this procedure relies on the use of an antibody that specifically and tightly binds its target protein in the buffer, and wash conditions used for the chromatin immunoprecipitation (ChIP) assay. Briefly, the protein–protein and protein–DNA complexes in vivo are reversibly crosslinked by formaldehyde. Specific antibodies are

From: *Methods in Molecular Biology, Vol. 285: Cell Cycle Control and Dysregulation Protocols*
Edited by: A. Giordano and G. Romano © Humana Press Inc., Totowa, NJ

then used to immunoprecipitate the protein targeted by the antibody from the cell lysate resulting in co-precipitation of DNA that was directly or indirectly crosslinked to that protein. Incubation at high temperature reverses the protein–DNA crosslinks to permit isolation and purification of the co-precipitated DNA that is subjected to polymerase chain reaction (PCR) analysis for establishing specific DNA sequences that are associated with proteins in vivo.

2. Materials

1. Phosphate-buffered saline (PBS).
2. Formaldehyde (37%).
3. Lysis buffer, 1% SDS, 10 mM ethylenediamine tetraacetic acid (EDTA), 50 mM Tris-HCl, pH 8.1.
4. Dilution buffer, 0.01% sodium dodecyl sulfate (SDS), 1.1% Triton X-100, 1.2 mM EDTA, 16.7 mM Tris-HCl, pH 8.1, 167 mM NaCl.
5. Sonicator.
6. Specific antibody against protein of interest.
7. Protein A/G Plus agarose beads (Santa Cruz).
8. Bradford assay reagent.
9. Low-salt buffer: 0.1% SDS, 1% Triton X-100, 2 mM EDTA, 20 mM Tris-HCl, pH 8.1, 150 mM NaCl.
10. High-salt buffer: 0.1% SDS, 1% Triton X-100, 2 mM EDTA, 20 mM Tris-HCl, pH 8.1, 500 mM NaCl.
11. LiCl buffer: 0.25 mM LiCl, 1% Nonidet P-40, 1% sodium deoxycholate, 1 mM EDTA, 10 mM Tris-HCl, pH 8.1.
12. Elution buffer: 1% SDS, 0.1 mM NaHCO$_3$. Do not keep longer than 1 mo.
13. 50-mL Screw cap tubes.
14. 1.5-mL Microcentrifuge tubes.
15. TE buffer.
16. 65°C Water bath.
17. Rotating wheel.
18. PCR reagents.

3. Method

1. Culture 2×10^6 cells on a 100-mm plate. If cell are grown in suspension, collect an equal cell number pellet by centrifugation.
2. Wash cells twice with 10 mL 1× PBS.
3. Add 10 mL of 1% formaldehyde diluted in PBS (1.35 mL of 37% formaldehyde to 50 mL) to crosslink the protein–protein and protein–DNA complexes in vivo. Incubate for 10 min at room temperature (*see* **Note 1**).
4. Wash twice with ice-cold 1× PBS.
5. Scrape cells in 10 mL of 1× PBS.
6. Collect cells by centrifugation at 4°C for 5 min (IEC centrifuge) at 500g.
7. Add protease inhibitors to lysis buffer.

8. Resuspend pellet in 0.3 mL of lysis buffer (0.3 mL per 100-mm plate) by pipetting up and down till pellet is thoroughly dispersed.
9. Incubate on ice for 10 min.
10. Sonicate samples for 10 s bursts. Rest for 30 s on ice and sonicate again for 10 s. Repeat at least three to four times. It is very important to keep the samples from warming up during sonication, which generates heat (*see* **Note 2**).
11. Centrifuge at 13,800*g* for 15 min in microfuge.
12. Transfer supernatant to a fresh tube and dilute 1:10 in dilution buffer.
13. Quantitate proteins by Bradford assay.
14. Use 1 mg of protein per ChIP reaction and add 1 μg of antibody per 200 μg of protein.
15. Rotate tubes gently for 1 h to over night at 4°C.
16. Add 10% v/v of A/G PLUS agarose beads.
17. Rotate tubes gently for 1 h at 4°C.
18. Centrifuge at 530*g* for 5 min at 4°C in a microfuge. Supernatant: unbound fraction; pellet (beads): bound fraction.
19. Save supernatant.
20. Wash beads with 1 mL of low-salt buffer.
21. Rotate tubes gently for 5 min at 4°C.
22. Centrifuge samples in a microfuge for 5 min at 530*g* at 4°C.
23. Wash beads with 1 mL of high-salt buffer.
24. Rotate tubes gently for 5 min at 4°C.
25. Centrifuge at 530*g* for 5 min at 4°C.
26. Wash beads with 1 mL of LiCl salt buffer.
27. Rotate tubes gently for 5 min at 4°C.
28. Centrifuge at 530*g* for 5 min at 4°C.
29. Wash beads with 1 mL of TE.
30. Rotate tubes gently for 5 min at 4°C.
31. Centrifuge at 530*g* for 5 min at 4°C.
32. Repeat step 29 through 31.
33. Add 250 μL of elution buffer.
34. Vortex at maximum speed for 10 s.
35. Rotate tubes gently for 15 min at room temperature.
36. Centrifuge at 530*g* for 5 min at 4°C.
37. Transfer supernatant to a clean microfuge tube.
38. To the pellet add 250 μL of elution buffer and repeat **steps 33–36**.
39. Combine supernatant with previous one.
40. Add 20 μL of 5 *M* NaCl or 3 *M* Na (oAc) to the combined eluted supernatants.
41. To the unbound fraction (from **step 18**), add 25 μL of 10% SDS per 500 μL of supernatant.
42. Reverse crosslinking by incubating tubes (containing bound and unbound fractions) at 68°C overnight.
43. Extract DNA with an equal volume of phenol-chloroform (25:24) mixture. Transfer aquas phase to a clean tube and extract DNA with equal volume of chloroform-isoamyl alcohol (24:1) mixture.

44. Centrifuge samples and transfer aquas phase to a new microfuge tube. Add 5-20 μg of glycogen as carrier and 0.9 volumes of isopropyl alcohol.
45. Precipitate DNA by centrifuging samples at 13,000 rpm for 15 min at 4°C.
46. Wash DNA pellet with 70% ethanol by centrifuging for 5 min as in **step 45**.
47. Air dry DNA pellet briefly and resuspend in 100 μL of 10 m*M* Tris-HCl ph 8.0.
48. Subject 3 mL of the eluted DNA to PCR using primer specific to gene of interest.
49. Resolve one-fifth of PCR product on agarose gel to determine the presence of amplified DNA region. Alternatively perform quantitative PCR using syber Green or fluorescently labeled probes.

4. Notes

1. The timing and temperature for optimal crosslinking varies for each transcription factor and cell type. We recommend optimizing conditions.
2. After sonication, the size of DNA fragment should be in the range of 100–1000 base pairs. Adjust the sonication conditions accordingly.

7

Protein–Deoxyribonucleic Acid Interactions Linked to Gene Expression

Electrophoretic Mobility Shift Assay

Amjad Javed, Sayyed K. Zaidi, Soraya E. Gutierrez, Christopher J. Lengner, Kimberly S. Harrington, Hayk Hovhannisyan, Brian C. Cho, Jitesh Pratap, Shirwin M. Pockwinse, Martin Montecino, André J. van Wijnen, Jane B. Lian, Janet L. Stein, and Gary S. Stein

1. Introduction

The electrophoretic mobility shift assay (EMSA) determines sequence-specific protein–deoxyribonucleic acid (DNA) interactions (e.g., transcription factors with cognate regulatory elements). This assay is based on reduced electrophoretic mobilities of protein/DNA complexes through a nondenaturing polyacrylamide gel compared with unbound DNA fragments or double-stranded oligonucleotides. If multiprotein complexes bind, the migration rate slows further with each additional protein. Oligonucleotide competition and antibody binding controls provide further evidence of binding specificity and protein identity. In competition experiments, unlabeled (cold) DNA or the same oligonucleotide (being used as a probe) with wild-type or mutated sequences of binding site or other unrelated binding sequences are added to the reaction. Interactions between the binding protein and the unlabeled related sequences would decrease the band intensity of the previously shifted complexes, whereas mutated or unrelated binding sequences will not change the intensity of the previously shifted complexes (an example is shown in **Fig. 1**).

To confirm the identity of the protein(s) interacting with the DNA sequences, the addition of antibodies that recognize the binding proteins to the reaction mixture produces an even slower migrating species than the original protein-DNA complex. This phenomenon is called a "supershift." If the antibody is

From: *Methods in Molecular Biology, Vol. 285: Cell Cycle Control and Dysregulation Protocols*
Edited by: A. Giordano and G. Romano © Humana Press Inc., Totowa, NJ

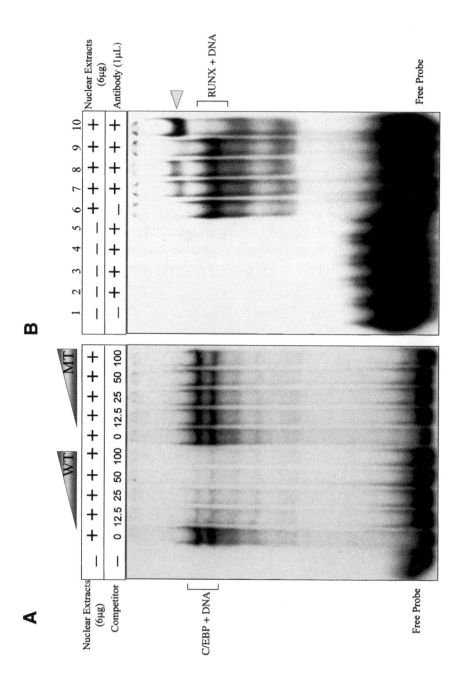

46

Fig. 1. Identification of regulatory protein interactions with promoter elements. Sequence-specific protein–DNA interactions were evaluated at the C/EBP site in the rat Osteocalcin promoter (**A**). Oligonucleotides (30 bp) representing wild-type (WT) and mutant (MT) sequences for C/EBP site were gel purified. WT probe was incubated with 6 µg of HeLa nuclear extracts and increasing concentrations (0, 12.5, 25, 50, and 100×) of either unlabeled WT or MT oligonucleotides. Formation of two closely migrating C/EBP specific complexes is indicated. Competition studies demonstrate sequence-specific protein–DNA binding, as the disappearance of complexes is observed only with the addition of WT but not MT competitors. RUNX proteins are the major component of the transcription factor complex binding to *Gallus* BSP promoter (**B**). Electrophoretic mobility antibody supershift analyses are shown for Gallus BSP promoter fragment containing recognition sequences for Runx factors. Nuclear extracts were pre-incubated with 1 µL of Runx antibodies for 20 min at 37°C followed by protein-DNA binding reaction (20 min at room temperature) with the addition of probe. Lanes 1 to 5 represent antibody controls for each site without nuclear extract indicating that antiserum alone does not react with the probe. Lane 6, the control, has 6 µg of nuclear extract without antibodies. Lanes 7–10 show the supershifts of the Runx complex with the Cbfβ, RUNX1, RUNX3, and RUNX2 antibody. The complex formed with ROS17/2.8 nuclear extract is completely supershifted in the presence of antibody specific to RUNX2/Cbfa1 (lane 10). Weak supershifts are also observed using antibodies specific to Cbfβ (a transactivator partner protein for Runx factors) and RUNX1 (lanes 7 and 8, respectively).

directed against the DNA binding domain of the protein(s), this will interfere and result in failure of the formation of the protein–DNA complex. This phenomenon is known as "blockshift." The addition of polypeptide (specific to the protein) in the reaction will also result in disappearance of the shift.

Key parameters that influence EMSA results are quality and purity of the transcription factor, binding conditions, gel running conditions, and the in vitro stability of protein–DNA complexes. The protocol described below is simple, relatively quick, and can be successfully used for a variety of transcription factors.

2. Materials

2.1. EMSA

1. Phosphate-buffered saline (PBS).
2. Nonidet-P40 (NP-40) lysis buffer: 1 mL of $1M$ Tris-HCl, pH 7.4, 300 µL of $1\ M$ MgCl$_2$, 1 mL of $1\ M$ NaCl, 500 µL of NP-40, water up to 100 mL. Filter sterilize (0.22 µm pore size filter) and store at 4°C.
3. Hypotonic buffer: 1 mL of $1\ M$ N-hydroxyethylpiperazine-N'-2-ethanesulfonate (HEPES), pH 7.9; 150 µL $1\ M$ MgCl$_2$, 1 mL of $1\ M$ KCl, water up to 100 mL. Filter sterilize (0.22µm pore size filter) and store at 4°C.

4. Extraction buffer: 2 mL of 1 *M* HEPES, pH 7.9, 150 µL of 1 *M* MgCl$_2$, 42 mL of 1 *M* KCl, 100 µL of 200 m*M* ethylenediamine tetraacetic acid (EDTA), 20 mL of 100% glycerol, and water up to 100 mL. Filter sterilize (0.22 µm pore size filter) and store at 4°C.
5. Complete protease inhibitor cocktail (Boehringer Mannheim). To generate 25× cocktail, dissolve one pellet in 2 mL of water. The solution is good for 14 d if stored at 4°C.
6. Coomassie protein assay reagent (Pierce, Rockford, IL).
7. KN100 buffer: 200 µL of 1 *M* HEPES, pH 7.9, 1 mL of 1 *M* KCl, 4 µL of 0.5 *M* EDTA, 2 mL of 100% glycerol, and water up to 10 mL. Store at room temperature.
8. Complementary oligonucleotides (400 ng).
9. Polynucleotide kinase buffer (1×) 70 m*M* Tris-HCl, pH 7.6, 10 m*M* MgCl$_2$, 10 m*M* dithiothreitol.
10. Bovine serum albumin (500 µg/mL).
11. [γ-^{32}P] ATP (100 µCi).
12. T4 polynucleotide kinase (10 U/µL; New England Biolabs, MA).
13. Water bath incubators.
14. Quick Spin Sephadex G-25 columns (Boehringer Mannheim).
15. Ecolume™ H solution (ICN, Costa Mesa, CA).
16. 1 *M* HEPES, pH 7.9.
17. 1 *M* KCl.
18. 1 *M* MgCl$_2$.
19. NP-40.
20. 0.5 *M* EDTA.
21. 1 *M* Tris-HCl, pH 7.4.
22. Nuclear extracts or purified protein.
23. Poly (dI-dC)·poly(dI-dC) (Roche). Dissolve 1 mg of powdered poly (dI-dC)·poly(dI-dC) into 1 mL of water. Store at –20°C.
24. Acrylamide: bisacrylamide solution (40:0.5). Dissolve 40 g of acrylamide and 0.5 g of bisacrylamide into 50 mL of distilled water by stirring for 20–25 min. Increase the volume to 100 mL by adding distilled water. Store in a dark bottle at 4°C.
25. Loading dye (0.25% [w/v] Bromophenol Blue, 0.25% [w/v] xylene cyanol, 40% [w/v] sucrose, dissolve in distilled water). Pass solution through a 0.22 µm filter and store at 4°C.
26. 10 × TBE buffer.
27. Glass plates, spacers, and comb.
28. Gel retardation apparatus.
29. Power supply.

3. Method

3.1. EMSA

3.1.1. Isolation of Nuclear Proteins

1. Grow cells to confluency in two to three 100 mm plates.
2. Aspirate media and wash cells with 10 mL of ice-cold PBS.

3. Keep plates on ice and scrap cells in 10 mL of ice cold PBS or collect 0.5 to 1 × 10^6 cells by centrifugation if in suspension.
4. Collect cells by centrifugation at 500g in an IEC centrifuge for 5 min at 4°C.
5. Resuspend cell pellet in 1 mL of ice-cold PBS and transfer to a prechilled Eppendorf tube.
6. Spin for 20 s at 200g at 4°C and drain carefully.
7. Resuspend cell pellet in 400 µL of ice-cold NP-40 lysis buffer by gentle pipetting with 1 mL tip. If the cell pellet is large, increase the volume of lysis buffer proportionally.
8. Incubate tubes on ice for 10 min.
9. Spin samples for 30 s at 200g in a microfuge at 4°C.
10. Gently but thoroughly resuspend the pellet in 400 µL of ice-cold hypotonic buffer (10 mM HEPES, pH 7.9, 1.5 mM MgCl$_2$, 10 mM KCl, containing protease inhibitor) as in **step 7**.
11. Collect the nuclei by centrifuging the samples at 4000g for 1 min at 4°C.
12. Resuspend nuclei pellet in 50–100 µL of ice-cold extraction buffer as in **step 7**. The nuclei pellet should be homogeneously suspended, increase the volume of the extraction buffer if necessary.
13. Vigorously rock the tubes in cold room for at least 30 min to 1 h.
14. Centrifuge samples at 8000g for 5 min at 4°C.
15. Transfer supernatant to a clean prechilled Eppendorf tube and aliquot nuclear extract in 20–25 µL per tube. Quick freeze aliquots in liquid nitrogen and immediately store at –80°C (*see* **Notes 1–3**).

3.1.2. Determination of Protein Concentration by Bradford Assay

1. Dilute 5 mL of Coomassie protein assay reagent (Pierce, IL) with an equal volume of distilled water.
2. Aliquot 1 mL of diluted Coomassie protein assay reagent into Eppendorf tubes.
3. Dispense known amounts of bovine serum albumin (2, 5, 10, 15, and 20 µg) to be used as standard.
4. Add 2, 4, and 6 µL of nuclear extracts to the 1 mL of diluted Coomassie protein assay reagent.
5. Determine the absorbency at 595 nm.
6. Plot the standard and the sample values to extrapolate the protein concentration (*see* **Note 4**).

3.1.3. End-Labeling of Oligonucleotide Probes (see **Note 5**)

1. Put 200 ng of gel purified top strand oligo into a clean Eppendorf tube.
2. Add 5 µL of 10× T4 polynucleotide kinase buffer (New England Biolab).
3. Add 5 µL of bovine serum albumin to a final concentration of 50 µg/mL.
4. Add 10 µL of [γ-^{32}P] ATP (100 µCi).
5. Add 2 µL of T4 polynucleotide kinase (10 U/µL).
6. Make up volume to 50 µL with nuclease free distilled water.

7. Mix the content carefully and incubate at 37°C for 1 h.
8. Add 400 ng of bottom strand oligo to the reaction mixture.
9. Boil at 100°C for 10 min.
10. Remove the beaker carrying tube and slow cool to room temperature for hybridization of the two strands (approx 45–60 min).
11. Briefly spin the tube and place on ice (*see* **Note 6**).
12. Equilibrate G25 column by centrifuging at 800*g* for 2 min.
13. Apply 50 µL of reaction to the center of column.
14. Collect flow through containing labeled DNA by spinning at 800*g* for 5 min.
15. Determine the specific activity (CPm/µL) of the labeled probe by adding 2 µL probe into the scintillation vial containing 4 mL of Ecolume™ H solution and measure in scintillation counter.
16. Labeled probe can be stored at 4°C for 2 wk or at –20°C for 3 to 4 wk.

3.1.4. Preparation and Prerunning of the Gel

1. Thoroughly wash two glass plates for vertical slab gels (Hoefer Scientific, CA) with 70% ethanol. Also clean two 0.75-mm spacers and Teflon comb with 70% ethanol and dry (*see* **Note 7**).
2. Assemble the gel sandwich on a clean surface. Lay down one glass plate first. Place the two 0.75-mm spacers along the edge of this plate. Place the second glass plate on top, grasp the glass plate sandwich and gently slide it into the clamp assembly.
3. Place the clamp assembly into the alignment position on the casting stand. Loosen the top screws to allow the plates and spacers to sit flush against the base and retighten the clamp screws.
4. Prepare a 4% gel by adding 4 mL of acrylamide: bisacrylamide (40:0.5) solution into a clean glass beaker.
5. Pipet 2 mL of 10× TBE buffer into the beaker.
6. Add 33.8 mL of distilled water and mix gently.
7. Freshly prepare 0.5 mL of 10% APS and dispense 200 µL into the solution.
8. Add 20 µL of TEMED, mix and immediately pour the solution into the glass plate sandwich with the help of a 10-mL pipet.
9. Place a 0.75-mm Teflon comb into the layer of gel solution (*see* **Note 8**).
10. Let the gel polymerize for 45–60 min at the room temperature.
11. Remove the comb carefully and flush the wells thoroughly with distilled water to clear any unpolymerized acrylamide.
12. Add 3 L of 1× TBE buffer in lower reservoir of the Hoefer vertical slab gel unit and place it on a magnetic stirrer stand.
13. Place the upper chamber unit on top of the gel plate assembly, clamp it tightly and fill it with 400 mL of 0.5× TBE buffer.
14. Transfer the upper chamber-gel plate assembly into the lower chamber and prerun the gel at 150V for 20–40 min (*see* **Note 9**).

3.1.5. Protein–DNA Binding Reaction (see ***Notes 10–14***)

1. Using guidelines in **Table 1**, label 0.5-mL tubes and dispense appropriate amounts of reagents.
2. To minimize pipetting errors, the components that require similar amounts may be combined as a master mix and then dispensed into individual tubes.
3. Assemble all the components of the binding reaction first and then add the DNA-binding protein (nuclear extract, purified proteins, and so on).
4. Incubate the reaction at room temperature for 20 min (*see* **Note 15**).

3.1.6. Electrophoresis of DNA–Protein Complexes

1. Turn off the power and remove the gel plate assembly. Fill the wells with 1× TBE buffer.
2. Load each binding reaction into the appropriate well of the pre-run gel using protein electrophoresis tips (Bio-Rad, Hercules, CA).
3. Load 20 µL of 2× loading dye into a separate well. The dye will be used to monitor the progress of electrophoresis (*see* **Note 16**).
4. Clamp the upper chamber on top of the gel plate and fill it with 400 mL of 1× TBE.
5. Run sample at 200 V for 1.5–2 h at 4°C. Stop the gel before the Bromophenol Blue approaches the bottom of gel (*see* **Note 17**).
6. Remove the gel plates from the chamber and remove carefully the side spacers.
7. Slowly pry the gel plates apart, allowing air to enter between the gel and glass plate (*see* **Note 18**).
8. Lay the glass plate with the gel attached on the bench with the gel facing up. Place a sheet of Gel Dryer filter paper (Bio-Rad) cut to size on top of gel. Carefully lift the paper from one end with the gel attached to it.
9. Cover the gel with plastic wrap and dry under a vacuum at 80°C for 30–45 min.
10. Expose the dried gel to X-ray film for 2–4 h (with intensifying screen) at –70°C or overnight without an intensifying screen.

4. Notes

1. Do not freeze thaw extracts more than three times or store in refrigerator.
2. Repeated freeze thaw cycles render the protein biologically inactive.
3. Save an aliquot for determination of protein concentration.
4. Generally, the expected yield of nuclear protein will range between 1.5–4 µg per µL with this protocol. The amount of extracted protein depends upon the salt concentration in the extraction buffer. It is important to note that if nuclear protein or transcription factor of interest is not detected or detected in low amounts, it might be because of less stringent extraction conditions. For optimal extraction of some nuclear factors, a higher salt concentration (this protocol uses 420 mM KCl) may be required. Alternatively, the DNA-binding factor can be obtained by in vitro transcription-translation or can be expressed in bacteria as glutathione *S*-transferase— fusion proteins. However, recombinant protein isolated in this way may not bind to

Table 1

A. Binding and Competition

	WT					MT				
	0X	12.5X	25X	50X	100X	0X	12.5X	25X	50X	100X
Nuclear extracts (2 µg/µL)	5 µL	5 µL	5 µL	5 µL	5 µL	5 µL	5 µL	5 µL	5 µL	5 µL
KN 100	5 µL	5 µL	5 µL	5 µL	5 µL	5 µL	5 µL	5 µL	5 µL	5 µL
Poly (dI-dC)·poly (dI-dC) (2 µg/µL)	0.5 µL	0.5 µL	0.5 µL	0.5 µL	0.5 µL	0.5 µL	0.5 µL	0.5 µL	0.5 µL	0.5 µL
Competitor (100 ng/µL)	–	1:4 / 0.5 µL	1:4 / 1 µL	1:4 / 2 µL	1 / 1 µL	–	1:4 / 0.5 µL	1:4 / 1 µL	1:4 / 2 µL	1 / 1 µL
Probe (40,000 cmp/µL)	1 µL	1 µL	1 µL	1 µL	1 µL	1 µL	1 µL	1 µL	1 µL	1 µL
Distilled water	8.5 µL	8 µL	7.5 µL	6.5 µL	7.5 µL	8.5 µL	8 µL	7.5 µL	6.5 µL	7.5 µL

Brackets: {Nuclear extracts, KN 100, Poly (dI-dC)·poly (dI-dC)} = 10 µL; {Competitor, Probe, Distilled water} = 10 µL (+ 20 µL dye).

B. Binding and Immunoshift

	WT					MT				
	0X	12.5X	25X	50X	100X	0X	12.5X	25X	50X	100X
Nuclear extracts (2 µg/µL)	–	1 µL	1 µL	1 µL	1 µL	5 µL	1 µL	1 µL	1 µL	1 µL
Antibody (100 ng/µL)	–	1 µL	1 µL	1 µL	1 µL	–	1 µL	1 µL	1 µL	1 µL
KN 100	10 µL	9 µL	9 µL	9 µL	9 µL	5 µL	4 µL	4 µL	4 µL	4 µL
Poly (dI-dC)·poly (dI-dC) (2 µg/µL)	0.5 µL	0.5 µL	0.5 µL	0.5 µL	0.5 µL	0.5 µL	0.5 µL	0.5 µL	0.5 µL	0.5 µL
Probe (40,000 cmp/µL)	1 µL	1 µL	1 µL	1 µL	1 µL	1 µL	1 µL	1 µL	1 µL	1 µL
Distilled water	8.5 µL	8.5 µL	8.5 µL	8.5 µL	8.5 µL	8.5 µL	8.5 µL	8.5 µL	8.5 µL	8.5 µL

Brackets: {Nuclear extracts, Antibody, KN 100, Poly (dI-dC)·poly (dI-dC)} = 10 µL; {Probe, Distilled water} = 10 µL (+ 20 µL dye).

The specific reagents required for gel retardation experiments are outlined. Generally, the reaction consists of two parts each in a 10 µL volume. The first component (DNA-binding protein) can be obtained from different sources (whole cell or nuclear extract, in vitro translated protein, bacterially expressed glutathione S-transferase–fusion protein, biochemical fractions). For "supershift" assays, antibodies are included. The second component of the reaction is the probe DNA. To avoid nonspecific binding of proteins to the probe, nucleic acid polymers are included [tRNA, sheared or restricted plasmid DNA, (poly(dI-dC), (poly(dG-dC), (poly(dA-dT)]. For competition assays, unlabeled specific and nonspecific DNA competitor are added. A positive and negative control reaction should be included with every experiment.

DNA like native proteins because of possible differences in post-translation modifications, such as phosphorylation or glycosylation, improper folding because of tag or prokaryotic environment, or the absence of co-factors, which may affect a binding protein's activity.

5. The purity of the oligonucleotides to be used as probe is of prime importance. We strongly recommend polyacrylamide gel electrophoresis purification of oligos followed by ethanol precipitation. DNA fragments (containing regulatory sequence) larger than 100 base pairs (bp) can be successfully purified by phenol-chloroform extraction. However, the probe DNA should be less than 300 bp in length to achieve sufficient separation between the free and bound species in the gel.

6. The removal of unincorporated nucleotides from the DNA probe is a very important step. It improves the quality of gel shifts and prevents contamination of gel chambers because of faster migration of free nucleotide into the buffer during electrophoresis.

7. Loading dye such as Bromophenol Blue and xylene cyanol or residual detergent on glass plates may interfere with the protein–DNA interactions.

8. Make sure no air bubbles are present underneath the tooth edges of the comb because they will cause small circular depressions in the well after polymerization. This will cause distortion of the band shift during separation.

9. This prerun before loading the samples will help to push ahead any contaminant that may be present and can interfere in the protein–DNA complex. Heat generated because of high voltage (used to run the gel) may distort complexes. We recommend running gels at 4°C.

10. While the gel is prerunning, start the protein-DNA binding reactions by mixing components using guidelines in **Table 1A**. This table is for competition assay using a 12-well gel. There are two components (10 μL volume each) of the reaction mixture: DNA binding protein and the DNA. The amount of nuclear extracts required to see a band shift should be determined before performing the competition assay. We recommend a range of 0–10 μg of nuclear extracts be tested with DNA probe containing wild-type and mutated binding sequences. KN100 is used to make up the volume of the first component. The second part consists of probe DNA, nonspecific competitor [i.e., poly (dI-dC)·(dI-dC)]. This nucleic acid polymer is added to the reaction to reduce nonspecific binding of proteins to the radiolabeled DNA fragment. The optimum amount (usually between 0 and 100 μg/mL) of poly(dI-dC) added to a reaction should be determined empirically for each DNA binding activity. Other nucleic acids that can be used to reduce nonspecific binding include tRNAs, poly(dA-dT) and poly(dG-dC).

11. Nuclear extracts like most protein preparations will contain both specific and nonspecific DNA-binding proteins. Competition binding assays will assess the sequence specificity of the protein–DNA interactions. For a specific competitor, the same DNA fragment or double-stranded oligonucleotide (unlabeled) as the probe should be used. The nonspecific competitor can be essentially any fragment with an unrelated sequence but perhaps the best control competitor is a DNA fragment or oligonucleotide that is identical to the probe fragment except

for a mutation(s) in the binding site that is known to disrupt function and binding. For most transcription factors that exhibit high affinity binding to a target DNA sequence, a 10- to 100-fold molar excess of unlabeled probe will eliminate the radiolabeled complex.

12. Competition assays are also used to identify a protein that is present in a shifted band especially, if a probe encompassing the 5' flanking region of a gene (promoter) is used that contains several different recognition elements within its sequence and thereby gives rise to multiple–DNA complexes with different mobilities. Addition of a 100-fold molar excess of an oligonucleotide containing a known recognition motif (e.g., RUNX regulatory sequences) should eliminate the shifted band corresponding to RUNX–DNA complexes.

13. Competition assays can also be used to identify critical nucleotides in the binding site of a given transcription factor. A series of competition assays can be conducted using oligonucleotides that differ in a single nucleotide from that used to identify the binding protein. The failure of mutant probes to compete the shifted band will indicate the crucial nucleotides required for binding in the recognition element.

14. If oligonucleotides are used as competitor, they should be hybridized before use. To generate double-stranded oligonucleotide, take an equal quantity of top and bottom strand (e.g., 100 ng each), boil for 10 min and slow cool to room temperature (45–60 min) for efficient annealing.

15. For antibody supershift assays, incubate small amounts of antibody with the nuclear extracts for 15–30 min at room temperature or at 37°C or overnight at 4°C before the addition of the second component of the reaction (probe DNA). After the addition of probe and other ingredients, incubate the reaction at room temperature for 20 min for protein–DNA interactions to take place. The amount of antibody required to see a supershift depends upon the affinity of antiserum and the abundance of transcription factor in the cell type used to isolate nuclear proteins. A control antibody reaction (antibody with probe alone; *see* **Table 1B**) should be included in the assay because the salt and other proteins in the antibody preparation may nonspecifically affect stability or mobility of the protein–DNA complexes. The addition of antibody sometimes results in appearance of a new shifted band that may represent antibody–DNA complex. If a transcription factor is a multiprotein complex, or the same binding sequences are recognized by similar family members, super shift assays can be performed by addition of antibodies to individual subunits separately. Antibodies that recognize the transcription factor in immunoblotting may not necessarily work in supershift. This discrepancy is usually caused by the inability of antibody to recognize the native protein. The best alternative is to use another antiserum that recognizes a different epitope on the binding protein. Other solutions to consider are increasing the salt concentration in the binding buffer, adding low concentrations (0.01–0.5%) of nonionic detergents (e.g., Tween-20, NP-40, and Triton X-100) to the binding buffer or increasing the amount of antibody in the reaction. The specificity of an antibody supershift can further be confirmed with peptide competition. Mix peptide with nuclear extracts and incubate at 22–37°C for 30 min. Add antibody to the reaction and incubate

again at 22–37°C for 30 min. Finally, add the remaining components to the tube and conduct protein-DNA binding by incubating at room temperature for 20 min.

16. Do not add any dye to the reaction because the dye may interfere in the protein–DNA interaction.

17. Bromophenol Blue migrates at approximately the same position as a 70-bp DNA probe. For smaller probes, do not run the Bromophenol Blue to the bottom of the gel.

18. Prying the plates apart too quickly may tear the gel or cause it to stick to both plates. The gel should remain attached to only one plate.

8

Protein–Deoxyribonucleic Acid Interactions Linked to Gene Expression

DNase I Digestion

Amjad Javed, Sayyed K. Zaidi, Soraya E. Gutierrez, Christopher J. Lengner, Kimberly S. Harrington, Hayk Hovhannisyan, Brian C. Cho, Jitesh Pratap, Shirwin M. Pockwinse, Martin Montecino, André J. van Wijnen, Jane B. Lian, Janet L. Stein, and Gary S. Stein

1. Introduction

Mapping DNase I hypersensitive sites can often localize the control regions in a eukaryotic gene. It is generally believed that chromosomal regions with loose or more open conformation are sensitive to DNase I cleavage. By comparing the patterns of hypersensitive sites obtained by digestion of silent genes with those obtained when the genes are actively transcribed, regions that participate in gene regulation (either induction or suppression) can be identified. A major strength of this method is that it is an "unbiased" approach to characterize the location of control sequences for the regulation of a gene. A good example of the power of DNase I hypersensitivity mapping is the rat Osteocalcin gene. Osteocalcin gene expression is detected only in bone tissues and in fully mature osteoblasts. DNase I cleavage is not observed in the OC gene in non-bone tissues or in immature osteoblasts (where OC is not transcribed). However, two DNase I hypersensitive sites are detected in the OC gene in bone tissues and in mature osteoblasts where the gene is actively transcribed. The first DNase I region encompasses the basal promoter regions that contain regulatory sequences for the RUNX, C/EBP, activator protein-1, and TFIID transcription factors. The second DNase I hypersensitive domain is mapped to a region 0.5 kilobases upstream of the transcription initiation site. This region contains a vitamin D enhancer element and regulatory sequences for RUNX

From: *Methods in Molecular Biology, Vol. 285: Cell Cycle Control and Dysregulation Protocols*
Edited by: A. Giordano and G. Romano © Humana Press Inc., Totowa, NJ

Scheme for DNase I Digestion

Rat Osteosarcoma ROS 17/2.8 Cell Line (9 days after plating)
Treatment of cells with 10^{-8} M vitamin D_3 ,collection &
isolation of nuclei by dounce homogenization in RSB buffer

↓

Collection & quantification of isolated nuclei

↓

Digestion of 20 units of nuclei with DNaseI for 10 minutes at $20^{\circ}C$

| 0 | 1 | 3 | 5 | 10 | U DNaseI |

Volume =1ml

Stopping of reaction & digestion with RNase & ProteinaseK for 16 hours at $37^{\circ}C$

↓

Phenol-Chloroform-Isoamyl alcohol (25:24:1) extraction (1x)

↓

Chloroform-Isoamyl alcohol (24:1) extraction (2x)

↓

Ethanol precipitation & resuspension in TE buffer

↓

Digestion of 20μg DNA with BamHI to release 4.8kb of OC gene

↓

Phenol-Chloroform-Isoamyl alcohol extraction, Ethanol
precipitation, washing & quantitation

↓

Electrophoresis of 10μg DNA on 1.2%
agarose for 16 hours at 30V. Transfer to
membrane and southern blot analysis with
BamH-HindIII probe

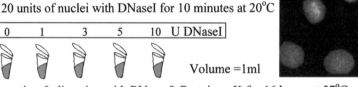

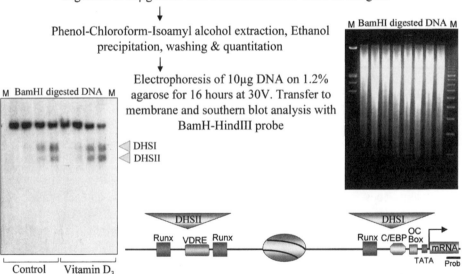

M BamHI digested DNA M

M BamHI digested DNA M

◁ DHSI
◁ DHSII

Control   Vitamin D_3

DHSII   DHSI

Runx VDRE Runx   Runx C/EBP OC Box

mRNA

TATA   Prob

◄───

Fig. 1. Schematic illustration of experimental procedure used for mapping DNase I hypersensitive sites. ROS 17/2.8 cells were cultured in 100-mm plates to confluency (when OC gene is actively transcribed). Cells were treated with 10^{-8} M vitamin D$_3$, 8 d after plating and collected 24 h later. Nuclei were isolated by dounce homogenization and an aliquot stained with DAPI (shown in figure at 63× magnification) to confirm their quality and cell lysis. Aliquots of 20 A$_{260}$units were digested with increasing concentration of DNase I for 10 min as indicated. DNA was then isolated by phenol-chloroform extraction, digested with indicated enzymes, and re-extracted with phenol chloroform. After electrophoresis in 1.2% agarose gel, DNA was transferred to a membranous solid support and hybridized with probes representing coding region of OC gene. A representative gel of digested genomic DNA along with markers (DNA digested with *Hind*III/*Eco*RI and 1-kb ladder) is shown. The probes were labeled by the random primer method using [α^{32}] P-dCTP and the Stratagene Prime-It II kit (Stratagene, La Jolla, CA). Hybridization was carried out at 65°C for 12 h with 1 ng of probe (10^{-9}cpm/μg specific activity) per 10-cm^2 membrane. The blots were analyzed by autoradiography or by using a STORM phosphorimager (Molecular Dynamics, Sunnyvale, CA). The appearance of two DNase I hypersensitive sites is indicated by arrowheads. The sensitivity of DNA to nuclease cleavage is greatly enhanced upon treatment of cell cultures with vitamin D$_3$ and runs parallel to increased OC transcription. The bottom panel shows a schematic representation of the OC promoter indicating the positions of binding elements for key transcription factors relative to the DNase I hypersensitive domains.

factors. The sequences at these hypersensitive sites are both sufficient and necessary for basal and bone-tissue specific expression of the Osteocalcin gene.

The most commonly used method of mapping a hypersensitivity profile involves the isolation of nuclei from a cell or tissue of interest followed by incubation of the intact nuclei with varying amounts of DNase I. An important control incubation is also included that contain no exogenous DNase I. The genomic deoxyribonucleic acid (DNA) from the treated and control nuclei is then purified by phenol-chloroform extraction and digested with a restriction enzyme. The fragments of DNA are resolved in agarose gels and southern blot analysis is performed with probes derived from the target gene (the scheme for DNase I digestion is shown in **Fig. 1**).

2. Materials

1. Phosphate-buffered saline (PBS).
2. RSB buffer: 10 mM Tris-HC1, pH 7.4, 10 mM NaCl, 3 mM MgCl$_2$.
3. Nonidet-40 (NP-40) RSB buffer: RSB buffer with 0.5% v/v NP-40.
4. Dounce homogenizer.

5. 0.4% Trypan Blue.
6. 4′, 6-Diamidino-2-phenylindole (DAPI 5 µg/µL).
7. Corex tubes.
8. Protease inhibitors.
9. Spectrophotometer.
10. DNase I (Worthington Biochemicals, Freehold, NJ).
11. 1 *M* CaCl$_2$.
12. Ethylenediamine tetraacetic acid.
13. 1% Sodium dodecyl sulfate.
14. RNase One (Promega, Madison, WI).
15. Proteinase K (Fisher Biotech, Fairlawn, NJ).
16. Buffered phenol.
17. Chloroform.
18. Iso-amyl alcohol.
19. 70% Ethanol.
20. TE buffer.
21. Microfuge.
22. IEC centrifuge.
23. Incubator.
24. Restriction endonuclease.

3. Method

3.1. DNase I Digestion

3.1.1. Isolation of Nuclei

1. Wash tissue culture plates with cold PBS twice.
2. Scrape cells in 10 mL of cold PBS.
3. Wash tissue culture plate with 10 mL of PBS and combine with previous one.
4. Collect cell pellet by centrifugation at 800*g* for 5 min at 4°C (IEC centrifuge).
5. Pour off the supernatant immediately.
6. Add protease inhibitors to NP-40 RSB buffer enough for the total volume, that is, including RSB buffer (*see* **Note 1**).
7. Resuspend pellet in 8 vol of cold NP-40 RSB buffer.
8. Transfer to a Dounce Homogenizer and using the loose pestle (B), give six to eight strokes on ice.
9. Add an equal volume of cold RSB buffer.
10. Transfer to a Corex tube.
11. Centrifuge at 300*g* for 5 min.
12. Add protease inhibitors to RSB buffer.
13. Pour off supernatant immediately.
14. Resuspend nuclei in 3–5 mL of cold RSB using a Pasteur pipet.
15. Evaluate cell lysis and integrity of isolated nuclei by staining an aliquot with 0.4% Trypan Blue 1:1 (v/v) or 4′, 6-diamidino-2-phenylindole (DAPI 0.5 µg/µL).
16. Measure A$_{260}$ of a 1:10 dilution (10 µL nuclei in 90 µL of room temperature RSB).

3.1.2. Digestion of Nuclei With DNase I

1. Digest 20 U of nuclei in 1 mL of RSB buffer (with protease inhibitor) containing 1 mM CaCl$_2$ with increasing concentrations of DNase I (normally ranges from 0–10 units) at room temperature.
2. Start the reaction by adding the nuclei.
3. Incubate samples at room temperature for 10 min.
4. Stop the digestion by adding ethylenediamine tetraacetic acid and sodium dodecyl sulfate to a final concentration of 25 mM and 0.5%, respectively.
5. Digest proteins by adding proteinase K to a final concentration of 200 µg/mL.
6. Incubate tubes at 37°C for 2–14 h.

3.1.3. Purification of Digested DNA

1. Add equal volume of phenol (pH 7.9) and chloroform:isoamyl alcohol (24:1) mixture to the reaction.
2. Rotate tubes gently at room temperature for 10 min.
3. Centrifuge samples at 900g in an IEC centrifuge at room temperature for 5 min (*see* **Note 2**).
4. Transfer aqueous phase to a new 15 mL phase lock tube.
5. Add equal volume of chloroform: isoamyl alcohol (24:1).
6. Rotate tubes gently at room temperature for 10 min.
7. Centrifuge samples at room temperature for 5 min at 900g in an IEC centrifuge.
8. Transfer aqueous phase to a clean Corex tube.
9. Add 1 µL of glycogen to each sample.
10. Add three volumes of 100% ethanol to each sample.
11. Mix gently and incubate tubes at –20°C for 10–15 h.
12. Precipitate DNA by centrifugation at 7300g for 50 min at 4°C.
13. Discard supernatant.
14. Wash pellets with 3 mL of ice-cold 70% ethanol.
15. Centrifuge at 7300g for 20 min at 4°C.
16. Pour off ethanol and let pellet dry at room temperature for 10 min.
17. Resuspend DNA in 300 µL of TE buffer.
18. Solubilize DNA by leaving tubes at room temperature for 2–15 h.
19. Transfer DNA to microfuge tubes and quantify by spectrophotometric analysis (*see* **Note 3**).

3.1.4. Restriction Digestion and Purification of the DNA

1. Digest at least 40–60 µg DNA with appropriate restriction enzyme(s) at 37°C overnight (use approx 5 U per µg of DNA).
2. Add 1 U of DNase-free RNase One (Promega) and incubate tubes at 37°C for 30 min.
3. Precipitate DNA by adding 1/10th volume of sodium acetate (3 M) and three volumes of 100% ethanol. Leave samples at –20°C for 2–15 h.
4. Centrifuge at 16,000g for 30 min at 4°C.

5. Wash DNA with 70% ethanol and centrifuge for 10–15 min as above.
6. Dry the pellet and resuspend in 50 μL of TE buffer.
7. Quantify the DNA and resolve 10 μg on 1% agarose gel for Southern blot analysis.

4. Notes

1. It is important to note that if protease inhibitors are included in the reaction, lesser amounts of DNase I should be used. As the cellular proteins will be preserved, including DNase I, an over digestion of the DNA might occur.
2. For an easy collection of the aqueous phase, we recommend using 15 mL Phase Lock Gel™ tubes (Eppendorf).
3. Because the isolated DNA is not RNA free, a high value of $A_{260/280}$ will be observed.

9

Protein–Deoxyribonucleic Acid Interactions Linked to Gene Expression

Ligation-Mediated Polymerase Chain Reaction

Amjad Javed, Sayyed K. Zaidi, Soraya E. Gutierrez,
Christopher J. Lengner, Kimberly S. Harrington, Hayk Hovhannisyan,
Brian C. Cho, Jitesh Pratap, Shirwin M. Pockwinse, Martin Montecino,
André J. van Wijnen, Jane B. Lian, Janet L. Stein, and Gary S. Stein

1. Introduction

Ligation-mediated polymerase chain reaction (LM-PCR) is used for high-resolution genomic footprinting. This technique was originally developed to study in vivo protein–deoxyribonucleic acid (DNA) interactions at regions of genes important for transcriptional regulation. Successful analysis of in vivo occupancy of gene regulatory elements by LM-PCR largely depends on the strategy and quality of reagents. The experimental outline for LM-PCR reaction is shown in **Fig. 1**. For a through understanding of this procedure and other alternative options, *see* Ausubel et al. *(1)*.

2. Materials

1. Phosphate-buffered saline (PBS).
2. First strand buffer 5×, 200 mM NaCl, 50 mM Tris-HCl, pH 8.9, 200 mM MgSO$_4$, 0.05% gelatin (*see* **Note 1**).
3. Loading buffer: 80% formamide, 45 mM Tris-HCl, 45mM boric acid, 1 mM ethylenediamine tetraacetic acid (EDTA), 0.05% Bromophenol Blue, 0.05% xylene cyanol.
4. Amplification buffer: 5× 200 mM NaCl, 100 mM Tris-HCl, pH 8.9, 25 mM MgSO$_4$, 0.05% gelatin, 0.5% Triton X-100 (*see* **Note 1**).

From: *Methods in Molecular Biology, Vol. 285: Cell Cycle Control and Dysregulation Protocols*
Edited by: A. Giordano and G. Romano © Humana Press Inc., Totowa, NJ

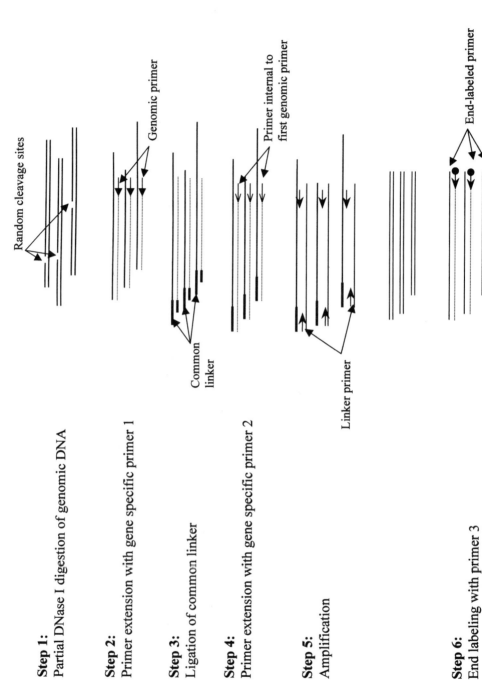

Step 1:
Partial DNase I digestion of genomic DNA

Step 2:
Primer extension with gene specific primer 1

Step 3:
Ligation of common linker

Step 4:
Primer extension with gene specific primer 2

Step 5:
Amplification

Step 6:
End labeling with primer 3

64

Fig. 1. Experimental outline for LM-PCR. The major steps involved in LM-PCR are schematically outlined. The cleaved genomic DNA is subjected to single-sided PCR, with a gene specific primer followed by ligation to a common linker. The ligated DNA is again subjected to a single sided PCR, with a second gene specific primer using processive polymerase such as Vent DNA polymerase. The last extension is conducted with an end labeled gene specific primer. The end-labeled extension products are visualized on a sequencing gel. Adapted from **ref. 2**.

5. Linker oligo mixture: 20 μ*M* oligonucleotide LMPCR-1 (5′-gcggtgacccgggagatct-gaattc-3′), 20 μ*M* oligonucleotide LMPCR-2 (5′-gaattcagatc-3′), 250 m*M* Tris-HCl, pH 7.7.
6. Thermocycler.

3. Method

3.1. Partial Digestion of Nuclei With DNase I

1. Isolate nuclei from the cells as described for DNase I footprinting.
2. Resuspend nuclei in RSB buffer without Nonidet-40 and estimate DNA concentration by absorption at 260 nm.
3. Digest aliquots of 20 A_{260} unit nuclei with increasing concentrations of DNase I (0 to 10 U, Worthington Biochemicals, Freehold, NJ) in a 400 μL final volume of RSB buffer with 1 m*M* $CaCl_2$ for 5 min at room temperature.
4. Stop the reaction by adding 400 μL of stop buffer (50 m*M* Tris-HCl, pH 7.5, 150 m*M* NaCl, 50 m*M* EDTA, 0.3% sodium dodecyl sulfate) and incubate with 1 U of RNase One (Promega) at 37°C for 1 h.
5. Extract samples once with phenol: chloroform, isoamyl alcohol (25:24:1) and once with chloroform, isoamyl alcohol (24:1) as described for DNase I digestion protocol.
6. Precipitate nucleic acids by adding 0.7 volumes of isopropanol.
7. Wash DNA pellet with 70% ethanol and resuspend in 100 μL of TE buffer.

3.2. Primer Extension and Ligation

For primer selection, *see* **Note 2**.

1. Perform primer extension in an automated thermal cycler under the following conditions: 95°C, 5 min; 62°C, 30 min; 75°C, 10 min (4 μg of DNA, 6 μL of 5× first strand buffer, 0.5 pg of primer 1, 0.24 μL of 25 m*M* dNTPs, 1 U of Vent DNA polymerase in a total volume of 30 μL; *see* **Note 3**).
2. Add 20 μL of ligase dilution mix (2 μL of 1 *M* Tris-HCI, pH 7.5, 0.35 μL of 1 *M* $CaCl_2$, 1 μL 1 *M* dithiothreitol, 0.25 μL of 10 mg/mL bovine serum albumin, 16.5 μL H_2O; *see* **Note 4**).

3. Add 25 μL of ice-cold ligase mix (5 μL of of 20 μ*M* linker, 2.5 μL of Promega ligase buffer, 0.5 μL of 100 m*M* ATP, 3 U of Promega ligase, or 100 U of NEB ligase, adding water up to 25 μL). Perform ligation at 16°C for 4–16 h.
4. Precipitate ligated DNA with ethanol and dissolve in 100 μL of water. Use 50 μL for single polymerase chain reaction

3.3. PCR

1. Add 40 μL of ice-cold amplification mix (18 μL 5× amplification buffer, 10 pmol long linker primer, 10 pmol primer 2, 0.8 μL 25 m*M* dNTP mix, H_2O up to 40 μL).
2. Transfer tubes to a preheated automated thermal cycler and add 10 μL of Vent mix (2 μL of 5× amplification buffer, 0.5 U of Vent DNA polymerase, and 7.5 μL of water).
3. Perform 18 cycles of PCR using following conditions (95°C for 1 min, 65°C for 2 min, and 76°C for 3 min).

3.4. 5′ End Labeling and DNA Purification

1. Perform 5′ end labeling of primer 3 (25pmol primer 3, 10 μL [γ-^{32}P] ATP, 2 μL of polynucleotide kinase, 5 μL of 10× polynucleotide kinase buffer, add distilled water up to 50 μL). Remove unincorporated ^{32}P by using G-50 columns (Amersham Pharmacia Biotech).
2. Add 10 μL of end labeling mix (2 μL of 5× amplification buffer, 2.5 μL of 1pmol per microliter of radiolabeled primer 3, 0.4 μL of 25 m*M* dNTP mix, 1 U of Vent DNA polymerase, adding water up to 10 μL) and perform two cycles of PCR (95°C for 4 min, 68°C for 2 min, and 76°C for 10 min).
3. Add 15 μL of stop solution (2.5 *M* sodium acetate, 50 m*M* EDTA).
4. Add 150 μL of phenol/chloroform and drop of phase-lock gel (Eppendorf) and mix by vortexing.
5. Microcentrifuge for 10 min and transfer upper layer to a new tube.
6. Add 5 μg of glycogen and 300 μL of 100% ethanol, mix, and chill for 30 min at –80°C.
7. Centrifuge and wash the DNA pellet with 70% ethanol.
8. Add 15 μL of loading buffer and denature samples 5 min at 85°C.

3.1.5. Denaturing Acrylamide Gel Electrophoresis

1. Load 7 μL of reaction on a 6% sequencing gel and resolve samples at 50 W.
2. Dry gel and analyze with a phosphorimager (Molecular Dynemics). Alternatively, the gel can be exposed to X-ray film for 14 h at –70°C.

4. Notes

1. Store buffer at –20°C.
2. For LM-PCR three gene-specific primers are required: primer 1 is for the extension reaction, primer 2 is for amplification, and primer 3 is for end labeling. It is helpful to design nested primers no longer than 27 base pairs with an increasing order of melting temperatures, that is, primer 1 with the lowest melting temperature and primer 3 with the highest melting temperature.

3. The amount of DNA used in this step is enough for two amplification reactions.
4. The addition of ligase dilution mix is to make first strand synthesis mixture compatible for T4 DNA ligase activity.

References

1. Ausubel, F. M., Brent, R., Kingston, R. E., et al. (2000) *Current Protocols in Molecular Biology*, John Wiley & Sons, New York, vol. 3, 15.5.1–15.5.26.
2. Mueller, P. R. and Wold, B. (1989) In vivo footprinting of a muscle specific enhancer by ligation mediated PCR. *Science* **246,** 780–786.

10

Assays for Cyclin-Dependent Kinase Inhibitors

Adrian M. Senderowicz

1. Introduction

Cyclin-dependent kinases (CDKs) are serine/threonine kinases that regulate cell cycle control and progression *(1,2)*. A CDK holoenzyme complex is active if associated with its cyclin partner and if the complex is phosphorylated at specific activating residues (threonine 160/161; **refs.** *1* and *2*). The progression through the cell cycle is mediated by the sequential activation of CDKs during different phases of the cycle. The G1/S phase transition of the cell cycle is mediated by phosphorylation of the Retinoblastoma gene product (Rb) by CDK4 and/or CDK6 (G1/ S checkpoint), leading to the release of bound E2F from Rb and allowing the transcription of genes by "free E2F" necessary for S-phase progression. During late G1 phase, the CDK2/cyclin E complex phosphorylates several substrates, including Rb. However, CDK2/cyclin A complex is active throughout the S phase. For cells to progress to mitosis, CDK1 (CDC2) must be "activated," and activated cdc2 phosphorylates substrates required for mitosis *(3)*.

Modulation of CDK function can be achieved by direct effects on the CDK catalytic subunit "direct CDK inhibitors" or by modulation of pathways necessary for the activation of CDKs "indirect CDK inhibitors" *(4,5)*. Examples of the first group include flavopiridol, UCN-01, paullones, hymenialdisine, roscovitine, and indirubins *(4–8)*. These compounds, when included in CDK *in vitro* kinases reactions (**Subheading 3.1.**), decrease the capacity of CDKs to phosphorylate its substrates.

In contrast, the indirect CDK inhibitors (such as rapamycin, lovastatin, antisense against CDKs, or cyclins) do not have the capacity, when included in CDK *in vitro* kinases reactions (**Subheading 3.1.**), to decrease the phosphorylation of CDK substrates *(4,5,9)*. However, these compounds could lead to loss in CDK activity in intact cells due to modulation of upstream pathways required

From: *Methods in Molecular Biology, Vol. 285: Cell Cycle Control and Dysregulation Protocols*
Edited by: A. Giordano and G. Romano © Humana Press Inc., Totowa, NJ

for CDK activation (**Subheading 3.1.**). Moreover, based on the known role of CDKs in the phosphorylation of specific endogenous substrates, we can assess the cellular effects of these compounds by Western blot using phospho-specific antibodies that recognize CDK-phosphorylated substrates (**Subheading 3.2.**). Finally, the block in cell cycle progression manifests the cellular consequence of CDK inhibition. This effect can be determined by the assessment of the DNA content as measured by FACS analysis (**Subheading 3.3.**).

2. Materials

All chemicals used should be of the highest quality and water should be deionized. Most reagents were obtained from Sigma. Mammalian cells are grown in a 5% CO_2 humidified incubator at 37°C and should be handled in sterile conditions at all times in a laminar flow-hood.

1. 1.5-mL Microfuge tubes.
2. 15-mL Centrifuge tubes.
3. 50-mL Centrifuge tubes.
4. Cell scraper.
5. 100-mm Cell culture plates.
6. 5-mL Polystyrene round-bottom tube.
7. Deionized water.
8. Absolute ethanol.
9. Phosphate-buffered saline (PBS): 37 mM NaCl, 2.7 mM KCl, 10 mM Na_2HPO_4, 1.4 mM KH_2PO_4, final pH 7.4.
10. β-Mercaptoethanol.
11. Dimethyl sulfoxide.
12. Ponceau S: 0.1% Ponceau S in 5% acetic acid.
13. Tween-20 (Sigma).
14. Tris-HCl, pH 7.4.
15. 0.5 M Ethylenediamine tetraacetic acid (EDTA).
16. 5-Bromo-2-deoxyuridine BrdU (50 mM stock in water, heat at approx 37°C to get into solution).
17. Rnase (Dnase free).
18. Propidium iodide: 50 µg/mL in PBS.
19. Gammabind G sepharose (Amersham).
20. Antirabbit and mouse IgG (Amersham).
21. Phospho-specific Rb antibodies (Cell Signaling Technology).
22. Enhanced chemiluminescent reagent (Amersham).
23. Bovine serum albumin (BSA).
24. Purified full-length Rb protein (QED Biosciences) or GST-Rb (Santa Cruz).
25. Histone H1 (Sigma).
26. Kinase lysis buffer (final concentration): 1 M N-hydroxyethylpiperazine-N'-2-ethanesulfonate, 0.5 M EDTA, 0.5% Nonidet P-40, 1 mM NaF, 10 mM β-glycerophosphate, protease inhibitor cocktail (200 mM sodium orthovanadate, 100 mM

dithiothreitol, 100 mM [4-(2-aminoethyl) benzenesulfonyl fluoride], 20 µg/mL aprotinin, 20 µg/mL leupeptin).

27. Kinase reaction buffer (final concentration): 50 mM N-hydroxyethylpiperazine-N'-2-ethanesulfonate, 10 mM $MgCl_2$, 5 mM $MnCl_2$, 2.5 mM ethylenebis(oxyethylenenitrilo)tetraacetic acid, 0.4 mM sodium vanadate, 10 mM β-glycerophosphate, 1 mM NaF, 1 mM dithiothreitol, cold ATP: 50 µM for CDK 1/2 assays and 5 µM for CDK 4/6 assays.

28. Immunoblot washing buffer (20×): 1 M Tris-HCl, pH 7.5, 50 mM EDTA, 1 M NaCl. Add 0.1% (v/v) Tween-20 after diluting the buffer to 1×.

29. Electrophoresis buffer: 25 mM Tris, 192 mM glycine, bring pH to 8.3 and then add 0.1% sodium dodecyl sulfate (SDS may damage the electrode).

30. Transfer buffer: 25 mM Tris-HCl, 192 mM glycine, and 20% methanol.

31. Kodak Bio-Max MR autoradiography film.

32. Autoradiography cassette.

33. PhosphorImager screen (Amersham).

34. Saran Wrap.

35. Whatman filter paper.

36. PVDF immunoblotting transfer membrane (Millipore).

37. Paraformaldehyde (make fresh for each use): heat 1 g of paraformaldehyde in H_2O at 65°C for 15 min and then add a few drops of 10 N NaOH. Finally, add 5 mL of 10× PBS.

38. LDS/SDS sample buffer (4× Invitrogen; 2× SDS Quality Biological).

39. Mouse anti-BrdU (clone B44, Becton Dickinson).

40. Donkey anti-mouse IgG Cy3-conjugated antisera (Jackson Immunochemicals).

41. Vectashield mounting medium with DAPI (Vector Laboratories, cat. no. H-1200).

42. Precast Tris-glycine polyacrylamide mini-gels (Invitrogen).

43. Antibodies against CDK1 (Life Technologies), CDK2, CDK4, and CDK6 (Santa Cruz).

44. Purified active CDK1/cyclin B1 (Life Technologies), active CDK2/cyclin A (Upstate Biotechnology).

45. Gel electrophoresis unit (Invitrogen).

46. Immunoblot transfer unit (Hoefer TE 22 Mini Tank Transphor Unit, Amersham).

47. Poly-D-Lysine (Roche).

3. Methods

3.1. Measuring CDK Activity In Vitro

Kinase assays are conducted with endogenous kinase from immunoprecipitated cells (**Subheading 3.1.2.**) or directly with recombinant-purified kinase (*see* **Note 1**).

3.1.1. Lysis of Mammalian Cells

1. Plate cells in 100-mm plates so that at the time of treatment the cells will be 50–60% confluent.

2. Harvest by washing twice with cold PBS and remove all residual PBS.
3. Add 100–250 μL of lysis buffer to 100-mm plates and scrape cells to one side.
4. Collect lysate in microcentrifuge tubes and continue lysis for 15 min.
5. Clarify lysate by centrifugation at 12,000*g* for 20 min to remove insoluble debris. Remove lysate to another microfuge tube without disturbing pellet.
6. Make protein standard with 1 μg/μL BSA. Aliquot and store at –20°C.
7. Prepare protein standard reagent (Bio-Rad protein assay reagent 1:5 v/v with water).
8. Add 2-, 4-, 5-, 7.5-, 10-, and 15-μg proteins to 3 μL of lysis buffer for standard curve. Sample protein lysate should be in the range from 2–4 μg/μL. Analyze with 3 μL of lysate in duplicates.
9. Read at 595 nm on a spectrophotometer.

3.1.2. Immunoprecipitation

1. Lyse cells and determine the protein concentration as in **Subheading 3.1.1.**
2. Use 200–500 μg proteins for the immunoprecipitation and 1–3 μg of antibody for 1 h at 4°C on a rotator.
3. Capture antibody by adding 25 μL of Gammabind G Sepharose for 30 min while rotating, wash twice with lysis buffer containing 100 m*M* NaCl for CDK 1/2 and 500 m*M* for CDK 4/6. Centrifuge at 13,000*g* for 3 min between each wash to pellet beads. Remove and discard supernatant with a pipet tip connected to a vacuum without disturbing beads.
4. Wash once with kinase buffer for the final wash.

3.1.3. In Vitro CDK Assay

Because this assay requires the use of radioactivity, care must be taken to limit your exposure and to prevent contamination of the laboratory. Always keep proteins at 4°C. Avoid freeze and thaw of proteins due to loss in kinase activity.

1. To the pelleted beads (or to purified recombinant CDK/cyclins), add 25 μL of kinase reaction buffer (*see* **Subheading 2, step 27**).
2. If a chemical compound being tested is dissolved in dimethyl sulfoxide, the concentration should not exceed 0.01% of the reaction mixture.
3. Add 50 μ*M* adenosine triphosphate (ATP) for CDK 1/2 or 5 μ*M* ATP for CDK 4/6; 10 μCi of {γ-^{32}P} ATP (300 Ci/mmol) to the reaction. Add as substrate for CKD 1/2 assays: 2 μg Histone H1, and for CKD 4/6 assays, 1 μg of full-length Rb (*see* **Notes 2** and **3**).
4. Incubate for 30 min at 30°C with shaking. Terminate by adding 4% SDS sample buffer. Heat sample at 95°C for 5 min.
5. Resolve samples by polyacrylamide gel electrophoresis, 8% for Rb and 12% for Histone H1.
6. Set power supply to 100 V and stop before dye front runs off gel. Remove gel from electrophoresis unit and place on filter paper. Cover with Saran Wrap.
7. Dry gel with a gel dryer for 45 min to 1 h at 80°C.
8. Expose film to autoradiography film and/or phosphorimager screen.
9. Develop film in film developer and/or phosphorimager (*see* **Fig. 1**).

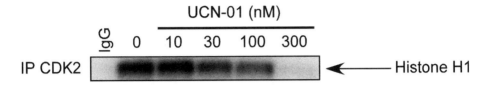

Fig. 1. In vitro CDK kinase assays. HN12 squamous head and neck carcinoma cell line were treated with the CDK inhibitor UCN-01 for 24 h, harvested, and kinase assay performed as shown in **Subheading 3.1.** As a control for specificity (negative control), unrelated IgG was used in place of the CDK2 antibody for the immunoprecipitation. The substrate used in the kinase reaction is Histone H1. Clear dose-dependent loss in H1 phosphorylation is shown.

3.2. Measuring CDK Activity in Intact Cells by Using PhosphoSpecific Antibodies Against Endogenous CDK Substrates

If a chemical compound inhibits CDKs in vitro, then it will be necessary to determine the phosphorylation status of the CDK substrate. Thus, either direct or indirect small molecule CDK inhibitors should lead to loss in the phosphorylation of endogenous substrates such as Rb, vimentin, NPAT, or p70S6 kinase (**refs. *10–14*;** *see* **Fig. 2**).

3.2.1. Polyacrylamide Gel Electrophoresis

1. Prepare protein lysate to a concentration of 1 µg/µL.
2. Add proteins to SDS sample buffer (5% β-mercaptoethanol for 2× sample buffer or 10% β-mercaptoethanol for 4× sample buffer) and add lysis buffer up to 25 µL.
3. Heat sample at 95°C for 5 min. Cells should be lysed and the protein concentration determined as in **Subheading 3.1.1.**
4. Add proteins to SDS sample buffer (5% β-mercaptoethanol for 2× sample buffer or 10% β-mercaptoethanol for 4× sample buffer) and add lysis buffer up to 25 µL.
5. Heat sample at 95°C for 5 min.
6. Load samples on to a 4–20% gradient or 8% Tris-glycine polyacrylamide mini-gel.
7. Initially set power supply to 100 V and then after 15 min increase the voltage to 150 V.
8. Saturate polyvinylidene diflouride (PVDF) membrane in methanol for 1 min and then in Tris-glycine buffer for 5 min.
9. Remove gel and place into Tris-glycine buffer.
10. Set up sandwich from transfer unit. First, place cassette in transfer buffer; secondly, place filter paper on sponge; third, place gel on to filter paper; fourth, place PVDF on to gel; fifth, remove any bubbles from underneath membrane; sixth, place wet filter paper on to membrane; seventh, place sponge on to filter; and lastly, close sandwich cassette and place into transfer unit.

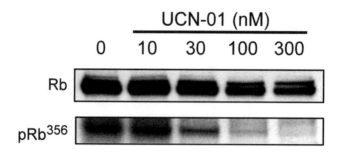

Fig. 2. Determination of CDK activity by Western blots against phospho-Rb antibodies parallel lysates from **Fig. 1** were run in SDS gel and immunoblotted as described in **Subheading 3.2.** In the upper band, an antibody recognizes total Rb levels and in the lower band, an antibody that recognizes only the phosphorylation of Rb at a CDK2 phosphorylation site, threonine[356] *(10)*. Clear dose-dependent loss in Rb phosphorylation is shown.

11. Transfer should be performed at 4°C at 80 V for 2 h or at 15 V for approx 15 h.
12. Remove membrane from transfer unit.
13. Wash membrane in PBS.
14. Check transfer efficiency and protein loading by Ponceau S staining for 1 min.
15. Rinse with PBS to observe protein staining.
16. Wash out the Ponceau S stain with TNE wash buffer for a few min.

3.2.2. Immunoblotting

1. Block PVDF membrane with 4% milk in TNE (*see* **Subheading 2., step 29**) for overnight at 4°C or for 30 min at room temperature while rocking.
2. Rinse once with TNE buffer.
3. Incubate with primary antibody for 1 h at room temperature or for overnight at 4°C while rocking.
4. Rinse once with TNE.
5. Wash membrane twice for 5 min each time with TNE.
6. Incubate with HRP-conjugated secondary antibody for 30 min at room temperature while rocking.
7. Rinse once with TNE.
8. Wash membrane twice for 5 min each time with TNE.
9. Incubate with ECL reagent for 1 min.
10. Expose film. Determine optimal exposure of film.

3.3. Effects of CDK Modulation on Cell Cycle Progression

Small molecules that lead to loss in CDK activity should arrest cells at different phases of the cell cycle. One traditional method to determine the percentage of cells in each phase is by measuring DNA content by FACS analy-

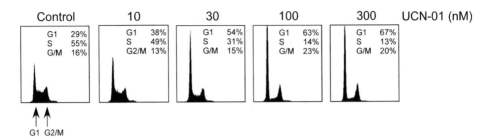

Fig. 3. Cell cycle analysis of UCN-01-treated cells by propidium iodide staining. Region between G1 and G2/M represents the S phase region.

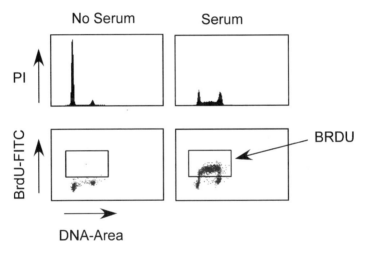

Fig. 4. BrdU and propidium iodide determination by FACS analysis. MCF10A breast immortalized cell lines were serum starved for 24 h (left panel) and then serum stimulated for 18 h (right panel). Upper panels represent propidium iodide labeling and lower panels represent BrdU incorporation. As shown in the upper panels, serum starved cells have 1% of S phase in comparison to serum (58%). Similarly, in the lower panels, serum starved cells have 1% of BrdU-positive cells compared with 57% of cells stimulated with serum.

sis (*see* **Fig. 3**). Also, the determination of S phase can be obtained by BrdU incorporation (DNA synthesis; *see* **Fig. 4**).

3.3.1. Assessment of DNA Content by Fluorescence-Activated Cell Sorting (FACS) Analysis With Propidium Iodide

1. Plate attached cells in 100-mm plates so that they are 40–50% confluent (approx 5 × 10^5 cells) upon treatment. For suspension cells, plate approx 4 × 10^5 cells/mL. At least 1 × 10^6 cells are needed for the assay.

2. Harvest attached cells by trypsinization for 3–5 min. Collect trypsinized cells with 4°C PBS. Centrifuge at 1000 rpm in a 15-mL tube. Suspension cells are collected directly into a 15-mL tube.
3. Wash once with PBS and centrifuge.
4. Resuspend pellet in 1 mL of PBS and add 4 mL of –20°C absolute ETOH. (Add ETOH in pulses of 1 mL each with repeater pipet while vortexing tube.)
5. Place samples at –20°C for minimum of 24 h and maximum up to 1 mo.
6. When sample is to be analyzed, centrifuge cells and remove ETOH. Wash once with PBS.
7. Resuspend cell pellet in 500 μL of 50 μg/mL propidium iodide solution in PBS plus 2 μg/mL RNAse without DNAse. Transfer to a 5-mL round-bottom tube.
8. Incubate for 1 h at 37°C. Analyze with a flow cytometer in the FL2 channel (*see* **Note 4** and **Fig. 3**).

3.3.2. Using FACS Analysis to Measure DNA Synthesis (S Phase) by BrdU Incorporation

1. Plate cells as described in **Subheading 3.3.1.**
2. Pulse cells with 50 μ*M* of BrdU 1 h before harvesting cells.
3. Follow **steps 1–6** from **Subheading 3.3.1.** on cell cycle analysis.
4. Slowly, add 500 μL of 2 *M* HCl/0.5% Triton X-100 a few drops at a time while maintaining a vortex. Incubate for 30 min at room temperature.
5. Centrifuge the cells at 1000 rpm for 5 min. Aspirate the supernatant and resuspend in 1 mL of 0.1 *M* $Na_2B_4O_7$. Centrifuge at 1000 rpm for 5 min.
6. Resuspend approx 10^6 cells in 1 mL of 0.5% Tween-20/1% BSA/PBS. Centrifuge at 1000 rpm for 5 min.
7. Add 300 μL of Tween/BSA/PBS and 20 μL of Anti-BrdU FITC. Incubate for 30 min at 37°C.
8. Centrifuge cells at 1000 rpm for 5 min. Resuspend in 1 mL of PBS containing 5 μg/mL propidium iodide.
9. Analyze on a flow cytometer. On a Becton Dickinson flow cytometer the FL1 channel will measure BrdU FITC and the FL2 channel will measure propidium iodide. Create a dot-plot and set the *X*-axis as FL2 and the *Y*-axis as FL1 (see **Fig. 4**).

3.3.3. Using Immunofluorescence to Measure DNA Synthesis (S Phase) by BrdU Incorporation

1. Autoclave glass cover slips and place into wells of six-well plate. Add 1 mL of poly-D-lysine to each well. Leave for 5 min and then wash once with PBS.
2. Plate approx 2×10^5 cells in each well.
3. Pulse cells with 50 μ*M* of BrdU 1 h before harvesting cells.
4. At harvest time, remove medium and wash once with PBS.
5. Fix cells in 2% paraformaldehyde for 20 min. Wash once with PBS. At this point, the cells may be stored at 4°C for up to 1 wk. Add 1 mL of Triton/BSA/PBS solution for 10 min.
6. Wash once with PBS containing calcium and magnesium. Add 100 U of DNAse I in 1 mL of Ca/Mg containing PBS for 1 h at 37°C.

7. Wash cover slips twice with PBS. Add 80 µL of 1:100 anti-BrdU in Triton/BSA/PBS solution to cover slip and incubate for 30 min at 37°C in a humidified chamber.
8. Wash twice with PBS. Add 80 µL of 1:500 anti-mouse conjugated Cy3 to cover slip for 30 min at 37°C in a humidified chamber.
9. Wash twice with PBS. Put one drop of mounting medium containing DAPI to a glass slide. After aspirating PBS from cover slip, carefully pick up cover slip with forceps and place down with the cells contacting the medium. The slides should be kept at 4°C in the dark until analysis for up to a week.
10. Stained cells can be visualized with a fluorescent microscope.

4. Notes

1. CDK1 (cdc2) kinase activity from endogenous sources: the number of cells with G2/M DNA content is low (15% total) in most exponentially growing cells, thus, the activity of cdc2 is quite low. In order to enrich cells with G2/M content (and active cdc2), aphidocolin-synchronized cells (arrested in S phase) can be released into media; and cells should be harvested approx 12 h later (depending on the cell line), when cdc2 becomes active.
2. It is important to mention that when comparing the inhibitory potency (IC$_{50}$ values) of different small molecule CDK inhibitors, the concentration of ATP in each reaction is of paramount importance as these small molecule CDK inhibitors compete with substrate (ATP). Thus, if the in vitro kinase reaction is performed with very high ATP concentrations, the potency is much lower than when the same compound is tested at lower ATP concentrations. Therefore, the only accurate way to compare these compounds is through the determination of a K_I with respect to ATP. This value is a constant and does not vary with ATP concentrations. For example, we can calculate the K_I app using this formula: $=IC_{50}/(1 + S/K_m)$, where S is the ATP concentration and K_m is the concentration of substrate (ATP) that leads to half-maximal velocity. If the ATP concentration used is lower than the K_m, then the IC$_{50}$ is similar to the $K_{i\ app}$ (**9**).
3. To determine whether a small molecule inhibits CDK activity by competition with ATP, kinase reactions should be done in the presence of increasing amounts of ATP while maintaining constant the amounts of kinase, substrate and inhibitor. Moreover, to determine if the inhibitor competes with substrate, increasing amounts of substrate should be tested in the presence of fixed amounts of kinase, ATP and inhibitor.
4. Set up a plot with the parameters: forward scatter on the *X*-axis and side scatter on the *Y*-axis. The second plot will be a histogram with FL-2 as DNA-Area. Fl-2 should be adjusted so that the G1 peak falls on channel 200 and then the G2/M peak will be at channel 400.

References

1. Morgan, D. O. (1995) Principles of CDK regulation. *Nature* **374**, 131–134.
2. Morgan, D. O. (1997) Cyclin-dependent kinases: engines, clocks, and microprocessors. *Annu. Rev. Cell Dev. Biol.* **13**, 261–291.

3. Sherr, C. J. (1996) Cancer cell cycles. *Science* **274,** 1672–6777.
4. Senderowicz, A. M. and Sausville, E. A. (2000) Preclinical and clinical development of cyclin-dependent kinase modulators. *J. Natl. Cancer Inst.* **92,** 376–387.
5. Senderowicz, A. (2000) Small molecule modulators of cyclin-dependent kinases for cancer therapy (review). *Oncogene* **19,** 6600–6606.
6. Hoessel, R., Leclerc, S., Endicott, J. A., Nobel, M. E., Lawrie, A., Tunnah, P., et al. (1999) Indirubin, the active constituent of a Chinese antileukaemia medicine, inhibits cyclin-dependent kinases. *Nat. Cell Biol.* **1,** 60–67.
7. Meijer, L. and Kim, S. H. (1997) Chemical inhibitors of cyclin-dependent kinases. *Methods Enzymol.* **283,** 113–128.
8. Meijer, L., Thunnissen, A. M., White, A. W., Garnier, M., Nikolic, M., Tsai, L. H., et al. (2000) Inhibition of cyclin-dependent kinases, GSK-3beta and CDK1 by hymenialdisine, a marine sponge constituent. *Chem. Biol.* **7,** 51–63.
9. Senderowicz, A. M. (2001) Cyclin-dependent kinase modulators: a novel class of cell cycle regulators for cancer therapy, in *Cancer Chemotherapy & Biological Response Modifiers* (Giaccone, G. G., Schilsky, R. L., and Sondel, P. M., eds.), Elsevier Science, Oxford, UK, Vol. Annual 19 (in press).
10. Kitagawa, M., Higashi, H., Jung, H. K., Suzuki-Takahashi, I., Ikeda, M., Tamai, K., et al. (1996) The consensus motif for phosphorylation by cyclin D1-CDK4 is different from that for phosphorylation by cyclin A/E-CDK2. *EMBO J.* **15,** 7060–7069.
11. Weinberg, R. A. (1995) The retinoblastoma protein and cell cycle control. *Cell* **81,** 323–330.
12. Zhao, J., Dynlacht, B., Imai, T., Hori, T., and Harlow, E. (1998) Expression of NPAT, a novel substrate of cyclin E-CDK2, promotes S phase entry. *Genes Dev.* **12,** 456–461.
13. Papst, P. J., Sugiyama, H., Nagasawa, M., Lucas, J. J., Maller, J. L., and Terada, N. (1998) Cdc2-cyclin B phosphorylates p70 S6 kinase on Ser411 at mitosis. *J. Biol. Chem.* **273,** 15,077–15,084,
14. Meijer, L., Borgne, A., Mulner, O., Chong, J. P., Blow, J. J., Inagaki, N., et al. (1997) Biochemical and cellular effects of roscovitine, a potent and selective inhibitor of the cyclin-dependent kinases cdc2, CDK2 and CDK5. *Eur. J. Biochem.* **243,** 527–536.

11

Protein Degradation Via the Proteosome

Henry Hoff, Hong Zhang, and Christian Sell

1. Introduction

It is becoming apparent that an increase in the rate of protein degradation represents one mechanism for the regulation of key proteins during the cell cycle (*1*). The importance of protein degradation in the control of cell proliferation is elegantly illustrated by the regulated synthesis and destruction of the cyclin family of proteins during the life cycle of a cell. The cyclins are a group of proteins that influence the function of a series of intracellular kinases (the cyclin-dependent kinases or CDKs). The activation of specific CDKs is required during specific phases of the life cycle of a cell (this life cycle is known as the cell cycle). For example, the longest phase of the life cycle of a cell is the phase known as G1, or gap 1, which precedes the replication of cellular deoxyribonucleic acid (DNA) during S phase. Cells in G1 contain relatively high levels of two cyclins, known as cyclin D and cyclin E. These two cyclins are degraded as cells enter S phase and begin to replicate their DNA. The orderly synthesis and degradation of the cyclins is critical to proper progression of cells through the phases of the cell cycle.

In addition to the regulation of the levels of cyclin proteins, protein degradation is involved in the regulation of a number of proteins important for cell proliferation and the list of proteins whose modes of regulation include some form of targeted degradation is steadily increasing. For the purposes of our discussion, we will focus on the regulation of a second messenger protein that is required for proliferation in response to insulin-like growth factor (IGF)-I. This protein, known as the insulin receptor substrate (IRS)-1, is phosphorylated by the activated IGF-I receptor and serves as a core for the assembly of a multiprotein complex at the plasma membrane. This multiprotein complex contains several proteins with known catalytic functions that regulate specific

From: *Methods in Molecular Biology, Vol. 285: Cell Cycle Control and Dysregulation Protocols*
Edited by: A. Giordano and G. Romano © Humana Press Inc., Totowa, NJ

responses within the cell. These catalytic proteins are known as second messengers, and the process of their activation by extracellular factors and the propagation of the signal to the nucleus is known as signal transduction.

Several lines of evidence suggest that the levels of IRS-1 within a cell dictate the response of a cell to IGF-I. In most cases cells will proliferate when exposed to IGF-I however, in specific settings, cells will differentiate in response to IGF-I exposure. For example, in muscle cell cultures low levels of IGF-I induce proliferation while higher levels of IGF-I induce differentiation. We have shown that the level of IRS-1 decreases in a dose dependent manner in epithelial cells exposed to IGF-I. This may explain the different response of muscle cells to IGF-I. In addition, the direct manipulation of IRS-1 levels in a hemopoietic cell line influences the decision of the cell to either proliferate or differentiate when exposed to IGF-I.

Recent work that we have performed *(2)* indicates that the IRS-1 protein is regulated primarily at the level of degradation. Specifically, the IRS-1 protein is targeted to the proteasome for degradation. This targeting involves the addition of ubiquitin moieties to the protein, a process that is thought to be a general mechanism for the targeting of proteins to the proteasome.

1.1. Regulation of Steady-State Protein Levels

Steady-state levels of any given protein are influenced by changes in the rate of synthesis and/or changes in the rate of degradation for that specific protein.

$$\text{Protein Abundance} = \text{Rate of Synthesis} - \text{Rate of Degradation}$$

After an observed change in the steady-state levels of a specific protein, both the rate of synthesis and the rate of degradation must be examined to determine whether one or both of these parameters has been altered to produce the observed change in protein levels. This chapter will outline procedures to initially examine the rate of synthesis of a specific protein as well as its rate of degradation.

Once it has been determined that the rate of synthesis of the protein under study is not the cause of the changes in steady state levels of the protein, one can begin to consider the possibility that the rate of protein degradation may be altered. In addition, the mechanism of the degradation of the protein must be considered. This chapter presents methods to examine the rate of synthesis and the half-life of a protein and also provides methods to examine the specific targeting of a protein to the proteasome. For recent reviews on the proteasome please (*see* **refs. *3*** and ***4)***. These methods are dependent upon the establishment that the protein of interest is indeed targeted to the proteasome under the conditions being studied. It must be remembered that there are multiple proteolytic pathways within a cell. The principle mechanisms for the degradation of proteins within the cell are proteasome mediated and lysosomal degradation. In our work we examined the degradation of IRS-1 and a series of specific inhibitors were used to determine if the protein was degraded via the proteasome or if another pathway was involved. Only inhibitors of the proteasome (lactocystin or MG132) had an effect on the degradation of IRS-1. Thus, we were able to focus on proteasome-mediated degradation as the likely mechanism for degradation of IRS-1. This type of approach is required prior to undertaking a detailed analysis of the ubiquitin conjugation of a protein.

1.2. [^{35}S]-Methionine Labeling

To quantitatively measure the synthesis or degradation of proteins, it is necessary to first label the protein of interest with a biosynthetic compound. In most circumstances, the label of choice is [^{35}S]-methionine. This chemical is available at high specific activity and is relatively simple to detect experimentally. Although methionine is not present in high abundance in proteins, it remains the most popularly used protein label. ^{35}S-cysteine can be substituted for [^{35}S]-methionine when the protein of interest contains few methionine residues (*see* **Note 1**).

The details underlying protein synthesis in mammalian cells are well documented *(5)*. Trans-labeled [^{35}S]-L-methionine is chemically indistinguishable from the free methionine available to the cell for protein synthesis. Thus, when trans label [^{35}S]-L-methionine is added to cells in the correct media, protein synthesis occurs as it would under normal circumstances. Activated tRNAs containing [^{35}S]-methionine are generated by aminoacyl-tRNA synthetase and ultimately incorporated into the growing polypeptide chain.

1.3. Rate of Synthesis

The rate of synthesis for a given protein can be measured by the amount of [^{35}S] methionine incorporation under standard growth conditions. This can be achieved by using a "pulse-chase" protocol (*see* **Note 2**). The protocol given is designed for adherent cells, but the same protocol can be used for nonadherent cells with several modifications (*see* **Note 3**).

1.4. Rate of Degradation

Protein half-lives in cells can vary from seconds to days. The half-life of a protein (the time it takes for 50% of a given protein to be degraded) is dependent on various conditions. For example, whether protein fragments are necessary to act as hormones or whether degradation of certain proteins is required for processes to occur (i.e., cyclin proteins), the state of the cell may affect the rate degradation of a given protein (again, the cyclin example is appropriate). The rate of degradation for a given protein can be determined by "pulsing" the cells with [^{35}S]-methionine following the method described in **Subheading 3.2.** and "chasing" the cells with excess unlabeled methionine at various time points. In this way the decrease in your labeled protein can be measured accurately over time. The protocol used for this pulse-chase analysis is identical to the protocol above with several modifications.

1.5. Mechanisms of Protein Degradation

As mentioned in **Subheading 1.1.**, the use of chemical inhibitors specific for intracellular proteolytic pathways can assist in the identification of the mechanism responsible for the destruction of a protein of interest. The use of these compounds will be dictated by the specific system that is being studied. For example, if a protein is degraded over a period of 32 h after the addition of a specific agent, then the protease inhibitors must be added for the entire time course and the levels of the protein of interest measured after the incubation period. The protocol given is tailored to the use of the proteasome inhibitor MG 132. An inhibition of protein degradation through MG132/lactocystin treatment will support the possibility that the protein is targeted to the proteasome. A negative result will indicate that the investigator must examine other proteolytic pathways for the degradation of the protein under investigation.

1.6. Immunoprecipitation and Western Blotting

To measure protein levels of your protein of interest, protein lysates are immunoprecipitated with a specific antibody and subsequently run on sodium dodecyl sulfate-polyacrylamide gel electrophoresis (SDS-PAGE). After SDS-PAGE, protein levels can be quantitatively measured or Western blotting can be performed to determine the relative level of your protein after treatment with various compounds, that is, MG 132 or lactocystin. This section presents protocols for the lysis of adherent cells, followed by immunoprecipitation of your protein of interest and finally a Western blotting protocol.

1.7. Quantitative Analysis

To accurately measure the rate of synthesis and/or degradation of a given protein, one must have the tools available to quantitate the results obtained from [^{35}S] incorporated protein lysates.

Because of the high specific activity of [^{35}S], SDS-PAGE gels can be exposed to X-ray film and images obtained in a short period of time (16–24 h). There are two commonly used methods to measure [^{35}S] protein incorporation after SDS-PAGE. In one case bands corresponding to your protein's appropriate size can be excised and counted using a scintillation counter. Another method is to scan the X-ray film using a phosphoimager or densitometer to obtain values for [^{35}S]-labeled proteins.

1.8. Transient Transfection of Adherent Cells

Once the investigator has determined the mechanism of degradation of their protein of interest (**Subheading 1.5.**), it may be necessary to transfect the modifying protein (in our case Ubiquitin) into the cells so that a high-enough level of the modified form of your protein is present to perform your studies. The protocol given is designed for adherent cells.

1.9. Conclusions

We hope that the techniques presented in this chapter will provide a resource for investigators who wish to explore the involvement of the proteasome in the regulation of a given protein. This set of procedures will allow the investigator to determine whether the proteasome or indeed, protein degradation, is involved the regulation of their protein of interest. We wish readers of this chapter the best of luck in their studies and hope that we have been able to provide some useful service.

2. Materials

2.1. Cell Culture

1. Cell culture media: sterile, is available from a variety of vendors. Media specific for the cell type under study should be used. Media should be stored at 4°C (*see* **Note 4**).
2. Sterile phosphate-buffered saline (PBS): 37 mM NaCl, 2.7 mM KCl, 10 mM Na$_2$HPO$_4$, 1.4 mM KH$_2$PO$_4$, final pH 7.4. Stable at room temperature.
3. Trypsin: sterile, available from a variety of vendors with or without ethylenediamine tetraacetic acid (EDTA). 10× solutions should be stored at –20°C until ready to use.

2.2. [^{35}S]-Methionine Labeling: Synthesis and Degradation

1. Complete cell-growth media: specific for the cell type, with the addition of 10% fetal bovine serum. Available from vendors, store at 4°C.
2. Methionine-free growth media: specific for the cell type, lacking methionine and no fetal bovine serum. Commercially available. Store at 4°C.
3. Trans label [^{35}S]-L-methionine >1000 Ci/mmol: available from vendors specializing in radiochemicals (i.e., NEN, ICN, Amersham) store at –80°C.
4. PBS: as described previously (**Subheading 2.1.**, **step 2**).
5. RIPA buffer: 50 mM Tris-HCl, pH 7.4, 1% Nonidet P-40, 0.5% sodium deoxycholate, 150 mM NaCl, 0.1% SDS, 1 mM ethylenebis(oxyethylenenitrilo)tetraacetic acid, 1 mM phenylmethyl sulfonyl fluoride, 1 μg/mL each aprotinin, leupeptin, pepstatin, 1 mM Na$_3$VO$_4$, 1 mM NaF.

2.3. Mechanism of Protein Degradation

1. Complete growth media: as described previously (**Subheading 2.2.**, **step 1**).
2. MG132: powder is available from Bio-Mol Corporation. This should be dissolved in dimethyl sulfoxide (DMSO).

2.4. Immunoprecipitation and Western Blotting

1. RIPA buffer: *see* **Subheading 2.2., step 5**.
2. Protein assay reagents: we prefer Pierce's Micro BCA Reagent Kit or Bio-Rad's Bradford Protein Assay Reagent. Both manufacturers provide protocols with the kit.
3. Protein A agarose: available commercially as a 50% slurry in PBS. Store at 4°C.
4. SDS-PAGE stock solutions and buffers: described in detail by Bio-Rad Gel Electrophoresis Manual (*see* **refs. 6** and **7**).
5. PBS: *see* **Subheading 2.1., step 2**.
6. Electroblotting buffers and apparatus: refer to same sources as mentioned for SDS-PAGE.
7. Primary and secondary antibodies: available from a variety of vendors. Individual antibodies are stored either at 4°C or –20°C.
8. 4× Laemmli sample buffer: for 8 mL, mix 3.8 mL of dH$_2$O, 1.0 mL of 0.5 M Tris-HCl, pH 6.8; 0.8 mL of glycerol, 1.6 mL of 10% SDS, 0.4 mL of 2-mercaptoethanol, and 0.4 mL of 1% Bromophenol Blue. Nitrocellulose: available from a variety of vendors, we suggest BA-85 Nitrocellulose from Schleicher and Schuell.
10. Carnation nonfat dry milk: available at local supermarket.
11. Western blotting detection reagents: chemiluminescent-based peroxidase specific reagents are available from a variety of companies. We recommend ECL reagents from Amersham, also NEN Renaissance Kit Works. These solutions are light sensitive and should be stored at 4°C.
12. X-ray film: we recommend Bio-Max MR film, which is available from a large variety of vendors.

2.5. Quantitative Analysis

1. X-ray film and film cassettes.
2. Phoshorimager or densitometer.
3. Scintillation counter and accessories.
4. Image analysis software.

2.6. Transient Transfection

As with the choice of culture conditions, the cell type will dictate the method of transfection that should be used. Transfection efficiencies vary widely in different cell types with a given transfection technique. There are numerous reagents commercially available for the transfection of mammalian cells, and the investigator should test a series of these on the cell type of interest. A list of transfection reagents and the commercial vendors that supply them is included below as a guide for the investigator. A cautionary note is in order however, this list is not meant to provide a comprehensive overview of transfection reagents. We urge the investigator to explore other vendors who may provide a reagent that better suits the specific application.

To optimize the transfection efficiency in the cell type to be studied and to monitor transfection efficiencies during individual experiments, we recommend the use of a reporter plasmid. If an inverted fluorescent microscope is available, a green fluorescent protein reporter plasmid is a good choice. Clontech provides a variety of fluorescent protein vectors that are suitable for this purpose.

The protocol given (**Subheading 3.8.**) is for transient transfection of adherent cells in 60-mm dishes and has been taken almost directly from the Superfect product literature. For transfections in other size dishes or flasks one should consult the protocol that comes with their transfection reagent of choice. These protocols will give the investigator the volumes of each solution to be used for a specific size flask. For our specific cell type, we found the Superfect reagent to give the highest transfection efficiency. The optimal agent must be determined empirically by the researcher for a given cell line.

3. Methods

3.1. Plating Cells

1. Wash cells with PBS. Add the PBS solution to the side of the plate to avoid disturbing the cell layer. The wash step removes serum proteins that inactivate trypsin and divalent cations that cells require for attachment to substratum.
2. Prepare a sterile trypsin-EDTA solution in a calcium- and magnesium-free salt solution such as PBS. The final concentration of trypsin in the solution should be 0.05% in calcium- and magnesium-free PBS. Addition of EDTA at 50 μM will aid in the detachment of some cell types but can be damaging to others. After removing the wash, add enough of the trypsin solution to cover the cell monolayer. We use 2 mL for a 150-mm flask and 1 mL for a 100-mm plate. Tip the plates to distribute the trypsin solution evenly. Place the plates in a 37°C incubator until the cells just begin to detach. Monitor the progress of the cells periodically under the microscope. Once the cells begin to detach, remove the trypsin solution and strike the sides of the culture vessel sharply with the palm of your hand to dislodge any adherent cells.
3. Add culture media containing serum to inactivate the trypsin and pipet the cell suspension vigorously to produce a single cell suspension. The cells should be transferred to a sterile polypropylene tube to prevent any cells from attaching to the culture dish while the cell number is determined.
4. Determine the cell number through the use of a hemocytometer or Coulter Counter.
5. Plate the cells at a density that will allow them to become approx 60% confluent on the day to begin your experiment. For our cells we use $2–3 \times 10^4$ cells/cm^2 to produce the proper cell density 24 h after seeding.

3.2. [^{25}S]-Methionine Labeling

1. Cells are grown to 60% confluence in complete media as described in **Subheading 3.1.**
2. Complete media is removed and cells are pulsed with 0.1–1.0 mCi/mL trans label [^{35}S]-L-methionine in methionine-free media for a period of time ranging from 10 min to overnight depending on the protein being investigated (*see* **Note 5**).
3. Media is removed, and cells are washed once with ice cold PBS.
4. Remove PBS, add 0.5 mL (100-mm dish) or 2 mL (T175 Flask) RIPA buffer to adherent cells and let rock at 4°C for 30 min.

5. Scrape lysed cells and pipet into 1.5-mL microcentrifuge tube.
6. Vortex tubes vigorously for 10–15 s, centrifuge at 4°C at 10,000g for 5 min.
7. Remove supernatant and place in new 1.5-mL microcentrifuge tube.
8. Perform Bradford or Pierce BCA Protein Assay (**Subheading 3.6.**).
9. Once protein concentrations are determined proceed to immunoprecipitation (**Subheading 3.6.**).

3.3. Degradation (Pulse-Chase)

Steps 1–3 are identical as in **Subheading 3.2.**

4. After PBS is removed, add complete media containing excess "cold" methionine (5–10 mg/mL). Place flasks in an incubator at 37°C, 5% CO_2 for various time intervals (*see* **Note 6**).
5. Remove media and wash once with ice cold PBS. Follow **steps 4–9** as in **Subheading 3.2.**

Once the protein concentrations are determined for the lysates prepared above, lysates are immunoprecipitated and separated by SDS-PAGE (**Subheading 3.6.**). The resulting gel can be quantitatively analyzed to determine the protein's rate of synthesis and degradation.

3.4. Inhibition of Proteasome-Mediated Degradation

1. Seed cells to achieve 50–60% confluence on the day of the experiment. The number of plates required is determined by the consideration of the appropriate controls. These include cultures treated to induce downregulation of the protein of interest and untreated controls in which the level of the protein of interest is unchanged. A dose response curve with a range of MG 132 is desirable. A good range would begin at 100 nM and end at 10 µM. Controls include a parallel series of cultures that receive DMSO alone. The MG132 dilutions should be prepared such that an equal volume of DMSO is added to each plate to ensure that there is no variation in protein level due to variations in DMSO concentration.
2. At 24 h after seeding (or when cultures achieve the desired density) place the cultures in complete growth medium containing MG132 for 15 min before the initiation of treatment to down-regulate the protein of interest. After this preincubation period, place the cultures into conditions that downregulate the protein of interest in the presence of MG132 or DMSO.
3. Incubate the cultures for the minimum amount of time required to achieve a clear downregulation of the protein of interest.
4. Lyse cells using RIPA buffer.
5. Determine protein concentration of samples.
6. Run SDS-PAGE and perform Western Blot analysis (**Subheading 3.6.**).

3.5. Protein Lysis of Cells

This protocol describes a method for the extraction of total cellular proteins from adherent cells. The same protocol can be used for cells in suspension cells, but cells are collected by centrifugation instead of being scraped.

1. After treatment with [^{35}S] or various compounds cells are removed from the incubator and placed on ice. Cells are washed three times with ice-cold PBS. After the last wash flasks should be tilted in a way such that all PBS is removed.
2. Add a specific volume of RIPA buffer or another lysis buffer of choice (*see* **Note 7**). Rock the flask containing cells and lysis buffer for 15–20 min at 4°C. After this time, using a cell scraper, scrape the lysed cells and remaining unsolubilized protein (*see* **Note 8**) to one side of the flask. Transfer the entire cell lysate into a microcentrifuge tube.
3. Sonicate the lysate (*see* **Note 9**) for 5 s and centrifuge at 11,000g for 5 min at 4°C.
4. Remove supernatant and place in new 1.5-mL microcentrifuge tube.
5. Perform a BCA or Bradford protein assay (*see* **Note 10**) to determine the concentration of total protein.

3.6. Immunoprecipitation

1. Dilute the cell lysate before beginning the immunoprecipitation to roughly 1μg/μL total cell protein with PBS in a microcentrifuge tube.
2. Add 4 μg of primary antibody (*see* **Note 11**) to 500 μg-1 mg cell lysate.
3. Gently rotate the mixture at 4°C overnight.
4. Add 40 μL of Protein A agarose and rotate the mixture for 2 h at 4°C.
5. Collect the pellet by centrifugation at 16,000g for 5 s.
6. Wash the pellet three times with PBS, each time repeating centrifugation as above.
7. After wash, spin down the pellet and discard supernatant. Add 40 μL of Laemmli sample buffer containing 2-mercaptoethanol to the agarose pellet and boil for 10 min.
8. Centrifuge at 11,000g for 5–10 s, load supernatant on SDS-PAGE gel, and perform electrophoresis (*see* **Note 12**).
9. After electrophoresis is complete, transfer the gel to nitrocellulose at 30 V overnight at 4°C (*see* **Note 13**).

3.7. Western Blotting

Depending on the antibody to be used the buffers used below may differ. Whenever the antibody is purchased, the supplier will send a protocol specific for that antibody. In general, either PBS or TBS is the buffer used, blocking is usually done with milk but BSA is sometimes recommended. One should consult the protocol given with their specific antibody and use this protocol as it is described. The protocol below is for an anti-IRS-1 polyclonal antibody in rabbit from Upstate Biotechnology (Lake Placid, NY).

1. After transfer, wash twice the nitrocellulose membrane with water.
2. Block the blotted nitrocellulose in freshly prepared PBS containing 3% nonfat dry milk for 20 min at room temperature or overnight at 4°C with constant agitation.
3. Incubate the nitrocellulose membrane with 0.5–1 μg/mL of primary antibody, diluted with freshly prepared 3% nonfat dry milk in PBS and rock at 4°C overnight (*see* **Note 11**).
4. Wash the membrane twice with water.

5. Incubate the nitrocellulose membrane in the secondary antibody (1:500–1:5000 dilution) for 1–2 h at room temperature (*see* **Note 11**).
6. Wash the nitrocellulose membrane twice with water and once with PBS-0.05% Tween once (10 min per each wash).
7. Rinse four to five times the nitrocellulose with water.
8. Use detection method of choice, expose to X-ray film, and develop.
9. Proceed to **Subheading 3.8.**

3.8. Quantitative Analysis

1. Protein samples isolated from cells that have been labeled with [^{35}S]-methionine are separated by SDS-PAGE and transferred to nitrocellulose as in **Subheading 3.7.**
2. After the transfer, the nitrocellulose filter is wrapped in plastic foil and exposed to X-ray film. For [^{35}S] blots, 1–2 d at –80°C should be sufficient. For Western blots, 30-s to 4-min exposure time is used depending on the antibody and relative level of expression of the protein (room temp).
3. Develop X-ray film.
4. One method to quantitate your [^{35}S]-protein bands is to excise the band from the nitrocellulose and count the amount of [^{35}S]-radioactivity using a scintillation counter. This is done by aligning your developed X-ray film with the membrane and marking the area (allow some extra space around the signal) with a ballpoint pen. Excise this area with a razor blade and place in 5- to 10-mL scintillation fluid. Count using a ^{35}S program. Remember to cut a "blank" square to record background. Make all excised squares the same size. After counting you will have a value (in cpm or dpm) for each protein square.
5. The other method used to quantitate X-ray film images (^{35}S or Western blot autoradiograms) is to scan the X-ray film itself. This is performed using a densitometer, phosphorimager, or other scanning device. In general, the higher the resolution of your scanning device (in pixels) the more accurate your measurement.
6. Once your X-ray film is scanned as in **step 5**, the image is loaded into a computer. Then it can be opened with an image analysis program. Once in the image analysis program, each protein band can be quantitated using boxes created around the signal. Again, it is important to create all the boxes the same size and to include a box with no signal as the background. The program will then give you a reading of the average density for that area (in pixels). In this way each protein band will have a value in pixels.
7. Once you have obtained values (cpm or pixels) for each of your protein bands, you are able to create a graph that will show values for each sample vs time. In this way one can get an estimate as to the relative rates of synthesis or degradation of the relevant protein over time.
8. When studying time-dependent processes (synthesis or degradation) it is critical to have equal amounts of protein at each time point. Without this, the results are not valid. We suggest that lysates (10–50 µg) be run separately on a SDS-PAGE gel and immunoblotted with an anti-beta-actin antibody or an antibody against a protein

whose levels do not change after stimulation of your cells. In this way you can make sure that the same amount of protein is being used for each time point.

3.9. Transient Transfection of Adherent Cells

1. The day before transfection, seed cells as in **Subheading 3.1.** The cell number seeded should produce 60% confluence on the day of transfection.
2. Incubate the cells at 37°C and 5% CO_2 in an incubator.
3. Dilute 5 µg of DNA (in our case, HA-Ubiquitin in an expression plasmid) dissolved in TE, pH 7.4 (minimum DNA concentration: 0.1 µg/µL) with cell growth medium containing no serum, proteins, or antibiotics to a total volume of 150 µL (*see* **Note 14**). Mix and spin down the solution for a few seconds to remove drops from the top of the tube (*see* **Note 15**).
4. Add 30 µL of SuperFect Transfection Reagent to the DNA solution (*see* **Note 16**). Mix by pipetting up and down five times or by vortexing for 10 s.
5. Incubate the samples for 5–10 min at room temperature (20–25°C) to allow complex formation.
6. While complex formation takes place, gently aspirate the growth medium from the dish and wash cells once with 4 mL of PBS.
7. Add 1 mL of cell growth medium (containing serum and antibiotics) to the reaction tube containing the transfection complexes (*see* **Note 17**). Mix by pipetting up and down twice, and immediately transfer the total volume to the cells in the 60-mm dishes.
8. Incubate cells with the complexes for 2–3 h at 37°C and 5% CO_2.
9. Remove medium containing the remaining complexes from the cells by gentle aspiration, and wash cells once with 4 mL of PBS.
10. Add fresh cell growth medium (containing serum and antibiotics). Incubate for 24–48 h at 37°C and then harvest cells as described. For example, cells transfected with HA-Ubiquitin are typically incubated for 24 h after transfection to obtain maximal levels of gene expression. After this time, cells can be treated with MG132 or Lactocystin to increase the levels of ubiquitinated proteins.

4. Notes

1. Trans label [^{35}S]-labeling products (i.e., ICN no. 51006) are available as a mixture of 70% [^{35}S]-L-methionine and 15% [^{35}S]-L-cysteine. This solution gives optimal in vitro labeling of cells. In the protocols given, the labeling solution is referred to as [^{35}S]-methionine. This is for simplicity. The actual solution to be used contains 15% L-cysteine with 70% L-methionine.
2. To measure the synthesis of a given protein, cells are "pulsed" with trans label [^{35}S]-L-methionine and then processed after a given time interval. To measure the rate of degradation for a given protein, cells are "pulsed" and subsequently "chased" with excess of nonradioactive methionine after various time intervals. The "chase" step is to abruptly stop ^{35}S incorporation and more accurately measure the degradation of the protein over time.

3. For nonadherent cells, cells are pelleted in a microcentrifuge tube at 5000*g* and washed by resuspension in PBS. This is in contrast to adherent cells that are washed directly in the flask. All other procedures can be used as in **Subheadings 3.2.** and **3.3.**

4. Cell culture conditions vary with the specific cell type used and the protocols should be modified to accommodate the cell type to be studied. In our studies, human prostate epithelial cells are used. These cells are propagated in a serum free medium that was developed by Gibco/Life Sciences for propagation of keratinocytes. It is worth noting that the composition of the media used should be carefully examined for any factors that may complicate the interpretation of the experimental results. The Keratinocyte serum free media from Gibco/BRL Life Sciences is provided as a technically serum free composition. However, the media is supplemented with bovine pituitary extract, epidermal growth factor, and high levels of insulin. The bovine pituitary extract is completely undefined so it is not clear what factors may be included in the culture medium or whether there is any advantage to this additive over the addition of fetal bovine serum. The addition of growth factors such as epidermal growth factor and insulin can alter cell responses dramatically and must be considered in the interpretation of any results if this medium is to be used. We have circumvented these difficulties by designing our experiments such that the cells are first shifted into a defined medium without additions to remove the complex mix of factors included in the media used for propagation. For an excellent guide to general tissue culture techniques, *see* **ref. 8.**

5. The time cells are "pulsed" varies widely and depends on the protein being investigated. Cyclins, for example, can be synthesized rapidly (10 min; **ref. 9**), whereas IRS-1 (a docking protein) needs overnight pulsing for detection *(2)*. The time one uses to pulse cells must be found empirically and depends entirely on the protein to be investigated.

6. When performing a pulse-chase experiment to investigate protein degradation, four to five flasks should be "pulsed" simultaneously. The plates are then "chased" by the addition of medium that contains an excess of unlabeled methionine to dilute out the labeled methionine and effectively stop the labeling. After desired time intervals (i.e., 0–4 h), one plate each should lysed as described using RIPA buffer. The times one chooses are dependent on the protein being studied and its relative rate of degradation.

7. The lysis buffer one chooses depends upon the protein being investigated. For our purposes IRS-1 can be well solubilized using RIPA buffer. Proteins present in the nucleus must be extracted using a nuclear extraction protocol as in *(6)*. Some proteins do not require such a harsh lysis buffer as RIPA buffer and lower amounts of detergents or salt can be used. For a review of lysis buffers, *see* **ref. 10.**

8. Depending on the lysis buffer, the time it takes for certain proteins to solubilize varies. We find that when using RIPA buffer, the nuclei remain on the plate even after 30 min; therefore, we scrape the nuclei and remaining lysate together.

9. Again, depending on the protein, different disruption techniques can be used. For example homogenization, vortexing, or we find sonication of the lysate gives optimal solubilization of IRS-1. We sonicate at 30 watts for 5 s on ice.

10. Bradford or BCA protein assays are based on proteins reacting with various compounds to emit a color change at a particular wavelength. The more protein the more color change at that wavelength. To perform an assay, a standard curve of a known protein and concentration (i.e., BSA 2 mg/mL) is diluted in a range from 2 to 40 µg. The lysates prepared are added separately (10–20 µL) in duplicate or triplicate and the color change is compared to the standard curve. It is of critical importance that this assay is done accurately, because when performing time course experiments equal amounts of protein must be used to obtain valid data.

11. Every antibody (monoclonal or polyclonal) purchased from a commercial vendor has a recommended amount (in µg/mL) to be used in immunoprecipitations. The same is true for Western blotting applications using primary and secondary antibodies. Usually, primary antibodies are diluted 1:500–1:2000, while secondary antibodies are diluted 1:200–1:5000 in the appropriate blocking solution. Each vendor should have this information available for the investigator.

12. For an overview of SDS-PAGE, one should consult the **refs. *6*** and ***7***. In general, for large proteins (>100 kDa) a 7.5% gel is used. For smaller proteins (<40 kDa) a 12.5% gel is run. Bio-Rad provides a very clear recipe for the buffers, and gel solutions used in SDS-PAGE in their electrophoresis manual that is provided when SDS-PAGE units are purchased.

13. For electrophoretic transfer of proteins one should consult the **refs. *6*** and ***7***. We transfer our gels at 60V for 2 h or 20 V overnight at 4°C.

14. Serum and antibiotics present during this step interfere with complex formation and will significantly decrease transfection efficiency.

15. The best results are achieved when plasmid DNA of the highest purity is used for transfection. DNA purified with QIAGEN and QIAfilter Plasmid Kits is ideally suited for transfection of most cell lines. For transfection of endotoxin-sensitive cells, we recommend using DNA purified with EndoFree Plasmid Kits. These kits efficiently remove bacterial lipopolysaccharide molecules during the plasmid purification procedure, ensuring optimal transfection results.

16. It is not necessary to keep SuperFect Reagent on ice at all times. 10–15 min at room temperature will not alter its stability.

17. At this stage serum and antibiotics no longer interfere with, but significantly enhance the transfection efficiency of SuperFect Reagent.

References

1. King, R. W., Desharies, R. J., and Peters, J. M. (1996) How proteolysis drives the cell cycle. *Science* **274,** 1652–1659.
2. Zhang, H., Hoff, H., and Sell, C. (2000) Insulin-like growth factor-I-mediated degradation of insulin receptor substrate-1 is inhibited by epidermal growth factor in prostate epithelial cells. *J. Biol. Chem.* **275,** 22,558–22,562.
3. Voges, D., Zwickl, P., and Baumeister, W. (1999) The 26S proteasome: a molecular machine designed for controlled proteolysis. *Annu. Rev. Biochem.* **68,** 1015–1068.
4. Hirsch, C. and Ploegh, H. L. Intracellular targeting of the proteasome. *Trends Cell Biol.* **10,** 268–272.

5. Lewin, B. (1997) *Genes VI*. Oxford University Press, New York, pp. 179–241.

6. Massachusetts General Hospital, Harvard Medical School. (1991) *Current Protocols In Molecular Biology*. John Wiley and Sons, New York, pp. 10.18.1–10.18.9.

7. Maniatis, T., Fritsch, E. F., and Sambrook, J. (1989) in *Molecular cloning: A laboratory manual* 2nd ed. Cold Spring Harbor Laboratory Press, New York.

8. Frechney, I. R. (1987) *Culture of Animal Cells: A Manual of Basic Technique*. Alan R. Liss, New York.

9. Sheaff, R., Singer, J., Swang, J., Smitherman, M., Roberts, J., and Clurman, B. (2000). Proteosomal turnover of P21[Cip1] does not require P21[Cip1] ubiquitination. *Mol. Cell* **5,** 403–410.

10. Harlow, E. and Lane, D. (1988) Immunoprecipitation, in *Antibodies: A Laboratory Manual*, (Ford, N., Nolan, C., and Ferguson, M., eds.), Cold Spring Harbor Laboratory, New York, pp. 421–470.

II

Analysis of the Factors Involved in Cell Cycle Deregulation

12

The Transformed Phenotype

Henry Hoff, Barbara Belletti, Hong Zhang, and Christian Sell

1. Introduction

Malignant tumors are composed of cells that have lost their proliferation control and multiply independently of a physiologic need for increase in cell number in the tissue. Cells that have lost these proliferative controls are often referred to as "transformed." Transformation of a mammalian cell has been defined as the acquisition of permanent disturbances of growth and/or locomotion control (1). This definition of transformation implies a phenotypic change that has been found to be induced either by the introduction of a new gene into a cell or by the mutation of the genome through either irradiation or deoxyribonucleic acid (DNA)-damaging agents. Genes that can be introduced into normal cells to produce a transformed phenotype are usually derived from oncogenic viruses. Thus the definition of transformation in mammalian cells differs form the definition of transformation in bacteria where the term refers to the introduction of any new gene into the bacterial genome.

The proliferative controls on cells in the body can be divided very roughly into two categories, a control on the maximal rate of proliferation and a control on the maximal number of cells within a given area. These parameters of proliferation are difficult to study in vivo, and in vitro systems have proven very useful for the study of various parameters of the transformed phenotype. The study of transformation in vitro began with the study of transforming tumor viruses. It was discovered in the 1970s that stromal cells infected with tumor viruses displayed altered growth characteristics in vitro. These altered characteristics included a loss of contact inhibition, reduced requirement for serum growth factors, and the ability to grow under conditions of anchorage independence. It was postulated that these changes reflected aspects of the

From: *Methods in Molecular Biology, Vol. 285: Cell Cycle Control and Dysregulation Protocols*
Edited by: A. Giordano and G. Romano © Humana Press Inc., Totowa, NJ

virus-induced phenotype that are important for tumor formation. This prediction was born out when a mutated form of the *Ras* gene was isolated from a human tumor by screening for changes in the in vitro growth characteristics of mouse fibroblast cells *(2)*. Since that time, the assay for altered growth characteristics in vitro has been widely used to study the transformed phenotype. In this chapter, we will describe simple assays to evaluate three characteristics of the transformed phenotype, contact inhibition, growth in reduced serum and anchorage independent growth. In addition, a protocol that describes a technique to study the survival of a nonadherent murine marrow cell line (32D cells) is given to illustrate how the transformed phenotype can be examined in suspension cultures. An excellent overview of the transformed phenotype can be obtained in Franks (1997) *(3)*.

1.1. Contact Inhibition and Growth in Reduced Serum

Contact inhibition refers to the fact that normal human stromal cells (such as fibroblasts or epithelial cells) when grown on a tissue culture dish will not grow on top of each other (fibroblasts will produce a multi-layer pattern in culture if given high levels of serum, but only at a very slow rate). Thus, a sparsely seeded population of cells will divide until they come into close contact with neighboring cells. At this time, their rate of division is greatly reduced even in the presence of growth factors or serum. Tumor (transformed) cells show no reduction in their rate of cell division at high densities. This is reflected in a higher yield of cells per unit area and the dividing cells are often shed into the culture medium. To illustrate this property of transformed cells, the researcher can perform a relatively easy proliferation (growth) curve over 7–10 d by counting total nontransformed and transformed cells in complete media. Performing the same experiment in 0.5–1.0% serum will illustrate how the transformed cell is able to divide rapidly with low serum levels.

Mammalian cells in culture rely on serum growth factors (such as the platelet-derived growth factor and insulin-like growth factors) for both survival and to stimulate cell division. As a rule, the serum derived from adult animals is relatively poor in these growth factors. Fetal serum derived from bovine fetuses has been widely used in tissue culture and the supplementation of a basal growth medium like Dulbecco's Modified Eagle Medium with 10% fetal bovine serum (FBS) will sustain the proliferation of most cell types. The expression of viral oncogenes reduces the cell's dependence on the presence of growth factors for cell division. The ability to grow in tissue culture medium supplemented with low levels of serum is a hallmark of virally transformed cells and can be measured by a simple growth analysis of the cells (as mentioned in the previous paragraph).

1.2. Colony Formation at Low Density

The cloning efficiency of a cell line refers to the ability of those cells to proliferate when plated at very low density such that each individual cell must divide without contact with other cells. Normal cells have a relatively low cloning efficiency (for human fibroblasts this efficiency is in the neighborhood of 1%). Transformed cells typically have a much higher cloning efficiency and the increase in cloning efficiency can be indicative of transformation. An estimation of the cloning efficiency of a cell line or cell strain can be determined by plating the transformed cell line at limiting dilutions, followed by staining with Crystal Violet dye.

1.3. Anchorage-Independent Growth

Normal stromal cells require substratum attachment to proliferate. This property is known as anchorage dependence and as the name implies, there is a requirement for attachment and some degree of spreading for cell division. The ability to proliferate under anchorage-independent conditions is a hallmark of transformation in fibroblasts and epithelial cells. The only cells that grow in suspension (i.e., in an anchorage-independent manner) are hemopoietic cells, transformed cells, or cell lines from malignant tumors. A simple and quantitative method for the assessment of the capacity for anchorage-independent growth in a cell line is the "soft agar" method. Although other methods are used, soft agar is a widely accepted method for the analysis of anchorage-independent growth.

1.4. Suspension Cultures: Survival of 32D Cells

Nonadherent (suspension) cell lines may also exhibit transformed properties. As an example of studies that may be performed on cells in suspension, we will describe survival studies of a myeloid cell line (32D), which is dependent on the presence of interleukin (IL)-3.

The 32D cell line is an IL-3-dependent myeloid cell line derived from normal murine marrow *(4)*. These cells have an absolute dependence for IL-3 and undergo apoptosis within 24 h after withdrawal of IL-3, even in the presence of 10% serum *(5)*. An important characteristic of this diploid murine hemopoietic cell line is that it expresses very low levels of insulin-like growth factor (IGF)-1 and insulin receptors and no insulin receptor substate (IRS)-1 or -2 *(6)*, whereas Shc proteins are strongly expressed. Overexpression of the IGF-IR in these cells prevents apoptosis caused by IL-3 removal upon IGF-I treatment and moreover induces a differentiation program along the granulocytic pathway *(7)*. Furthermore, if 32D cells overexpressing the type 1 insulin-like growth factor receptor (IGF-IR) are stably transfected with the IRS-1 cDNA, the cells no longer differentiate but instead grow indefinitely even in the absence of IL-3 when treated with IGF-I. Conversely, if 32D cells are stably transfected with a plasmid overexpressing the Shc protein, they rapidly differentiate *(7)*. It seems therefore that proliferation or differentiation of 32D IGF-IR cells depends on the availability of substrates, with IRS-1 promoting proliferation and Shc proteins favoring differentiation.

IGF-IR, when activated by its ligands, plays an important role in the growth of cells. Because it is mitogenic, it is quasi-obligatory for transformation and it can protect a cell from a variety of apoptotic injuries. The IGF-1R can also induce differentiation in certain types of cells *(8)*. The mechanism by which the IGF-IR switches from one signaling system to another is in itself of considerable interest and this switching phenomenon can be studied with relative ease by using the 32D cell line.

2. Materials

2.1. Contact Inhibition and Growth in Reduced Serum

1. Complete growth media: specific for the cell type, with the addition of 10% FBS. Available from a variety of vendors, sterile, store at 4°C.
2. Sterile phosphate buffered saline (PBS): 137 mM NaCl, 2.7 mM KCl, 10 mM Na$_2$HPO$_4$, and 1.4 mM KH$_2$PO$_4$. Bring pH to 7.4., stable at room temp.
3. Sterile trypsin: available from a variety of vendors with or without ethylenediamine tetraacetic acid (EDTA; *see* **Note 1**). 10× solutions should be stored at –20°C until ready to use. 10× trypsin is diluted 1 to 10 with PBS.
4. 6-, 12-, or 24-well sterilized tissue culture dishes.
5. Hemocytometer or Coulter Counter.

2.2. Colony Formation at Low Density

1. Complete growth media: as described in **Subheading 2.1., step 1**.
2. PBS: as described in **Subheading 2.1., step 2**.
3. Trypsin: as described in **Subheading 2.1., step 3**.
4. 0.5% Crystal Violet solution: 0.5 g of Crystal Violet dye in 100 mL of distilled H$_2$O. Sterility is not necessary.
5. Cell fixation solution: 50% methanol/50% acetic acid. For other cell fixation solutions, consult **ref. 9**.

2.3. Anchorage-Independent Growth (Growth in Soft Agar)

1. Complete growth media: as described in **Subheading 2.1., step 1**.
2. 2× Complete growth media: most commercial media comes in a powdered form with packages prepared in a way to make 1 L of 1× media. To make 2× complete media dissolve the contents in 500 mL of distilled H$_2$O and filter sterilize. Add fetal bovine serum to a final concentration of 20%.
3. 2% Agarose: 2 g of agarose in 100 mL of distilled H$_2$O.

4. 0.5% Agarose: 0.5 g of agarose in 100 mL of distilled H_2O.
5. PBS: as described in **Subheading 2.1.**, **step 2**.
6. 1× trypsin without EDTA: as described in **Subheading 2.1.**, **step 3**.
7. 6-Well or 60-mm sterile tissue culture plates.

2.4. Suspension Cells: Survival of 32D Cells

1. 32D Cells transfected with IGF-IR or with IGF-IR, and IRS-I.
2. 6-Well tissue culture plates.
3. Hank's balanced solution.
4. RPMI 1640 medium supplemented with 10% heat-inactivated fetal bovine serum and 2 mM L-glutamine.
5. IGF-I: 50 ng/mL (Life Technologies).
6. Trypan Blue (Life Technologies).
7. Hemocytometer.
8. Centrifuge for cytospin.
9. SureStain Wright (Fisher Diagnostics).
10. Giemsa Stain (Fisher Diagnostics).

3. Methods
3.1. Contact Inhibition and Growth in Reduced Serum

1. Grow cells to 70–80% confluence in complete growth media.
2. Wash cells twice with PBS (a volume equal to the volume of complete growth media the cells were grown in).
3. Add 1× trypsin without EDTA (a volume equal to half the volume of PBS added for the washings). Incubate cells 10–15 min. in a 5% CO_2 incubator at 37°C.
4. When cells are floating, add an equal volume of complete growth media and centrifuge for 5 min at 200–240g.
5. Remove supernatant and resuspend cells in 10–20 mL of complete growth media (*see* **Note 2**).
6. Count an aliquot of the cells using a hemocytometer or Coulter Counter. Dilute the cells to 1×10^4 cells/mL media.
7. Using 6-, 12-, or 24-well sterile tissue culture plates, seed at least 42 individual wells with 1×10^4 cells/cm^2 per well (*see* **Note 3**).
8. Place the plates into a 5% CO_2 incubator at 37°C.
9. The next day remove one plate each of transformed and nontransformed cells. Wash three wells of each plate three times with PBS (the volume of PBS should be equal to the volume of media used to seed the cells). Add 1× trypsin without EDTA (one third of the volume of PBS used for the washings) and replace in incubator for 10–15 min.
10. When the cells are floating, add an equal volume of complete media and pipet cells up and down thoroughly.
11. Count an aliquot of the cells or all the cells (*see* **Note 4**) and make your counts in triplicate.

12. Repeat **steps 9** to **11** each day for at least 7 d. The longer (in days) you perform these steps, the more accurate the saturation curve will look for each cell line (*see* **Note 5**).

13. After all counts are obtained, take the average of each day (along with standard deviations) and plot the cell number vs days in culture.

14. From the graph created in **step 13**, you should see a plateau (or equal numbers) after 5 to 7 d for the nontransformed cell line (*see* **Note 5**). The transformed cell line will not show this and the numbers should continue to increase over time. In this way, one can illustrate how a transformed cell line has lost its contact inhibition in comparison to the non-transformed cell line.

15. The same protocol as that above (**steps 1** to **14**) can be performed in low serum (0.5–1.0% FBS) to illustrate how a transformed cell line proliferates more than a nontransformed cell line in low serum conditions.

3.2. Colony Formation at Low Density

1. Cells are grown in complete media until 70–80% confluence.
2. Cells are trypsinized with 1× trypsin without EDTA in PBS until cells are floating. At this point, add an equal volume of complete growth media.
3. Centrifuge the cells for 5 min at 200–240g.
4. Resuspend cells in complete growth media as to give a concentration of $1–5 \times 10^5$ cells/mL. Count cells using a Coulter Counter or Hemocytometer (*see* **Note 2**).
5. Dilute cells to 1×10^2 cells/mL, 1×10^3 cells/mL, 1×10^4 cells/mL, 1×10^5 cells/mL with complete growth media. Only 2 to 5 mL of each dilution is needed.
6. Plate cells with complete growth media using 1 mL of each dilution and 10 mL complete growth media per plate. This is for 100-mm dishes. Use 0.3 mL of each dilution + 3 mL complete media for 60-mm dishes.
7. Allow cells to grow for at least 8 d or until colony formation can be seen (*see* **Note 6**).
8. Remove media and wash cells twice with PBS.
9. Add cell fixation solution (50% methanol/50% acetic acid) and fix cells for 15 min at –20°C.
10. Remove fixative and allow cells to air dry at room temperature by inverting the dish. Plates should be dry within 10 min.
11. Add 0.5 % Crystal Violet solution and stain cells for 5–10 min at room temp (*see* **Note 7**).
12. Place a large glass Pyrex dish in a sink and place the stained plates with the Crystal Violet solution on the plates facing up. Place a large beaker (1 L) in the middle of the Pyrex plate and turn water on so that it flows into the beaker steadily. The water will overflow out of the beaker and go into the plates. Allow this to continue for 20–30 min.
13. Colonies should be seen with the naked eye. The size of the colonies depends on the cell line being used. In any case, transformed cells will have a higher percentage (>20%) of colonies per plate as compared to nontransformed cells.

3.3. Anchorage-Independent Growth (Growth in Soft Agar)

1. Grow transformed and nontransformed cells to 70–80% confluence in complete growth media.
2. Make 2% agarose and 0.5% agarose solutions. Dissolve agarose completely in a microwave. When the agarose is dissolved, cover top of flask with aluminum foil and place the agarose solutions in a 50°C waterbath to keep the temperature of the agarose constant at 50°C.
3. Wash and trypsinize cells as in **Subheading 3.1.** Resuspend the cells at a concentration of 1×10^5 cells/mL in 1× complete growth media, as in **Subheading 3.2., steps 1** to **4**.
4. Calculate the number of six wells or 60-mm dishes you wish to use. You should have at least three wells for transformed and nontransformed cells. As an example, we will use one six-well plate for transformed cells and one six-well plate for non-transformed cells.
5. Each six-well plate or 60-mm dish will need 2 mL of bottom agarose. So, for one six-well plate you will need 12 mL of bottom agarose. Remove 2% agarose from 50°C waterbath and 2× complete growth media from 37°C waterbath. Add 7.5 mL of 2% agarose to 7.5 mL of 2× complete growth media, mix, rapidly pipet 2 mL of the solution into each well avoiding bubbles (*see* **Note 8**).
6. After agarose has solidified in the wells, calculate the number of wells you wish to plate. For a six-well plate, you will need 6×1.5 mL = 9 mL.
7. Remove 0.5% agarose from 50°C waterbath and 2× complete growth media from 37°C waterbath. Add 5 mL of 0.5% agarose to 5 mL of 2× complete growth media, mix, add 1 mL of cells diluted to 0.5×10^4 cells/mL in complete growth media. Mix well and rapidly pipet 1.5 mL of the solution to each of the wells avoiding the introduction of bubbles (*see* **Note 9**).
8. After upper layer has hardened (10–15 min), add 1.5 mL of complete growth media on top of agarose.
9. Place dishes into 5% CO_2 incubator at 37°C for approx 21 d (*see* **Note 10**).
10. View plates on an inverted microscope and focus up and down to observe colony formation. Colonies should be >150 µ to be counted (this can be determined using an ocular micrometer, which fits in the eyepiece of the microscope).
11. The transformed cell line should have many more colonies than the nontransformed cell line.

3.4. Suspension Cells: Survival of 32D Cells

1. Collect exponentially growing cells and wash them three times in HBS. Centrifuge at 500*g* for 5 min each time.
2. Resuspend the pellet in an appropriate volume of RPMI 1640 medium containing 10% heat-inactivated fetal bovine serum and 2 m*M* L-glutamine and count the cells.
3. Seed cells at a final concentration of 1×10^5 cells/2 mL medium/well in six-well tissue culture plates. Prepare six wells for each cell line to be tested: two wells

without IGF-1 will serve as negative control (since these cells will die within 48 h). In the remaining four wells, add IGF-1 50 ng/mL. Two wells will serve for the counting at d 4 (and for the replating of d 8), the other two wells will serve for the counting at d 6.

4. At d 2, check the cells for viability, but counting is not necessary.
5. At d 4 count the cells: transfer the 2 mL/well of cells in IGF-1 in a 15-mL Falcon tube, centrifuge 5 min at 500*g*, and resuspend in 2 mL of RPMI 1640 medium containing 10% heat-inactivated fetal bovine serum and 2 m*M* L-glutamine. In an Eppendorf tube, mix 100 µL of cells with 100 µL of Trypan Blue and count the cells with a hemocytometer. Cells are alive when they are capable to "exclude" Trypan Blue, so that dead cells will be blue, whereas alive cells will be white. When calculating the final number of cells, remember to include the dilution factor (1:2) used to prepare the cells with Trypan Blue.
6. At d 4 you will also need to replate cells in fresh medium for d 8. On the basis of the previous counting, replate 1×10^5 cells/2 mL medium/well from each "d 4 well" in RPMI 1640 medium containing 10% heat-inactivated fetal bovine serum, 2 m*M* L-glutamine, and IGF-1 50 ng/mL.
7. At d 6 and d 8 you will need to count the cells/well following exactly the same protocol used at day 4.
8. At d 4, 6, and 8: on the basis of the previous counting, take 7×10^4 cells and bring them to a final volume of 300 µL with PBS.
9. Prepare the cells in duplicate to have two slides per sample.
10. Cytospin at 500*g* for 10 min and let the slides dry at least a couple of hours before proceeding to the next step.
11. Add one drop of Surestain Wright on the cytospinned cells and allow to stand for 30 s.
12. Wash in deionized water.
13. Dilute Giemsa 1:10 in deionized water, add 1 drop to the slide, and allow to stand for 10 min.
14. Wash extensively in deionized water.
15. Let the slides dry completely before mounting the cover slip and observe them at the microscope.
16. Classify as "undifferentiated cells" those showing a blast or meta-blast morphology; classify as "differentiated cells" those showing a band morphology and polymorphonucleated cells.

4. Notes

1. Trypsin with EDTA is most useful for epithelial cells, whereas trypsin without EDTA is used for fibroblast cells.
2. Depending on the cell type and the density of the cells, the amount of media one uses to resuspend their cells will vary. As an estimate, a confluent 100-mm dish of fibroblast cells can be resuspended in 10 mL of 1× complete growth media after trypsinization. An aliquot of this resuspension should be counted using a hemocy-

tometer or Coulter Counter and then diluted in 1× complete growth media to the correct concentration.

3. To obtain accurate proliferation values for nontransformed and transformed cell lines, multiple counts (number of cells) should be done for each time point (we use three replicates each counted three times). To see the difference in proliferation between transformed and nontransformed cells, cells should be counted each day for at least 7 d. Thus, at least 21 wells are needed for each cell line.

4. Our cell counts are performed using a Coulter Counter. An aliquot of the cells can also be counted using a hemocytometer and the multiplying by the dilution factor.

5. Nontransformed cells will cease to proliferate when the number of cells reaches a high enough level (they exhibit contact inhibition). The number of days it takes for this to occur will vary with the cell type and cell line. This must be determined empirically (i.e., if the cell line being investigated takes 10 d to begin to plateau, then set up 30 wells for that cell line). Transformed cell lines will continue to proliferate even at high cell numbers (they are not contact inhibited).

6. Depending on the cell type and cell line, the amount of time it takes for an individual cell to form a colony will vary. Cells divide exponentially (i.e., 2-4-8-16-32); thus, if the doubling time for a certain cell line is 1 d, then after 7 d there should be 128 cells. Transformed cells will form colonies more rapidly then nontransformed cells. Colonies should be visible by sight after 10–12 d. This also varies with the cell line.

7. Crystal Violet dye stains proteins. After 5–10 min, the cells should be dark blue by sight. Longer staining is not necessary. If the cells are not blue, the dye solution should be checked or the fixative changed.

8. It is important not to have the agarose begin to solidify while pipetting. To avoid this, only mix enough 2% agarose with media to do three to four wells, then discard the pipet and repeat for each set of wells. Also, after removing the agarose solution from the 50°C waterbath, mix with the media quickly. If a problem arises, the agarose solution should be microwaved again and placed at 50°C.

9. When adding the 0.5% agarose solution, it is very important that the solution is not warmer then 50°C, otherwise cells will be killed. As in **Note 8**, prepare enough 0.5% agarose, media, and diluted cells to fill only three wells at a time and then repeat. If the agarose begins to harden too quickly, remicrowave the agarose, place at 50°C and repeat.

10. Depending on the cell type and cell line being investigated, the time it takes for colonies to form will vary. However, as a general rule, colonies should start to become visible using an inverted microscope after 2 to 3 wk. It is important to remember that the colonies form within the agarose and the microscope must be focused up and down to see the colonies at different levels within the agarose.

References

1. Ponten, J. (1976) The relationship between in vitro transformation and tumor formation in vivo. *Biochim. Biophys. Acta* **458,** 397–422.

2. Newbold, R. F. and Overell, R. W. (1983) Fibroblast immortality is a prerequisite for transformation by E. J. c-Ha-*ras* oncogene. *Nature* **304,** 648–651.
3. Franks, L. M. and Teich, N. M. (1997) *Introduction to the Cellular and Molecular Biology of Cancer,* 3rd ed. Oxford University Press, New York.
4. Greenberger, J. S., Sakakeeny, M. A., Humpries, R. K., Eaves, C. J., and Eckner, R. J. (1983) Demonstration of permanent factor-dependent multipotential (erythroid/neutrophil/basophil) hematopoietic progenitor cell lines. *Proc. Natl. Acad. Sci. USA* **80,** 2931–2935.
5. Valtieri, M., Tweardy, D. J., Caracciolo, D., Johnson, K., Mavilio, F., Altmann, S., et al. (1987) Cytokine dependent granulocytic differentiation. *J. Immunol.* **138,** 3829–3835.
6. Zhou-Li, F., Xu, S-Q., Dews, M., and Baserga, R. (1997) Co-operation of simian virus 40 T antigen and insulin receptor substrate-1 in protection from apoptosis induced by interleukin-3 withdrawal. *Oncogene* **15,** 961–970.
7. Valentinis B., Romano G., Peruzzi F., Morrione A., Prisco M., Soddu S., et al. (1999) Growth and differentiation signals by the insulin-like growth factor receptor in hemopoietic cells are mediated through different pathways. *J. Biol. Chem.* **274,** 12,423–12,430.
8. Baserga R., Hongo A., Rubini M., Prisco M., and Valentinis B. (1997) The IGF-I receptor in cell growth, transformation and apoptosis. *Biochim. Biophys. Acta* **1332,** F105–F126.
9. Harlow, E. and Lane, D. (1988) *Antibodies: A Laboratory Manual,* Cold Spring Harbor Laboratory, New York.

13

A Morphologic Approach to Detect Apoptosis Based on Electron Microscopy

Martyn K. White and Caterina Cinti

1. Introduction

Apoptosis, or programmed cell death, refers to both the initiation and execution of the events whereby a cell commits suicide. This process is important in development and its deregulation is found in many diseases *(1–6)*, including cancer *(6–10)*. Apoptosis is distinct from other ways in which cells may lose viability (e.g., necrosis, senescence). Apoptosis is an active process triggered by a variety of stimuli, which induces closely comparable structural changes (**Fig. 1**). These morphological changes are especially evident in the nucleus where the chromatin condenses to compact and apparently simple, globular, crescent-shaped figures *(11)*. Other typical features include cytoplasmic shrinkage, zeiosis, and the formation of apoptotic bodies within the nucleus. The earliest definitive changes in apoptosis that have been detected by electron microscopy are compaction of the nuclear chromatin into sharply circumscribed, uniformly-dense masses that abut on the nuclear envelope and condensation of the cytoplasm. Continuation of condensation is accompanied by convolution of the nuclear and cellular outlines, and nucleus often break up at this stage to produce discrete fragments. The surface protuberances then separate with sealing of the plasma membrane, converting the cell into a number of membrane-bounded apoptotic bodies of varying size in which the closely packed organelles appear intact; some of these bodies lack a nuclear component, whereas others contain one or more nuclear fragments in which compacted chromatin is distributed either in peripheral crescents or throughout cross-sectional area. The final step of apoptosis is characterized by massive cell hydration after cytoplasm membrane fragmentation and degraded within lysosomes of apoptotic bodies. Many assays are

From: *Methods in Molecular Biology, Vol. 285: Cell Cycle Control and Dysregulation Protocols*
Edited by: A. Giordano and G. Romano © Humana Press Inc., Totowa, NJ

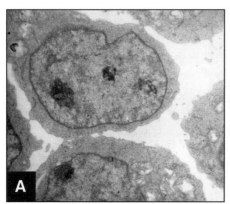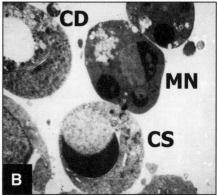

Fig. 1. (**A**) Normal-growing T-lymphoblastoid (CCRF-CEM) cells. (**B**) T-lymphoblastoid (CCRF-CEM) apoptotic cells at different phases of apoptotic response. Chromatin margination organized into cap-shaped (CS) electron-dense structure underlying the nuclear envelope, micronuclei (MN), and cell presenting cytoplasm membrane disintegration (CD). Kindly provided by Dr. Nicoletta Zini and Dr. Caterina Cinti, ITOI CNR, Bologna, Italy.

available to detect and measure apoptosis. Cells that enter apoptosis undergo a series of ultrastructural changes involving different nuclear domains at distinct phases (early and late) of apoptotic process and the electron microscopy technique is a sensible method to visualize either early or late morphological changes at high ultrastructural level (e.g., for early phase: chromatin margination firstly limited to tin electron-dense areas underlying the nuclear envelope and secondly organized into cap-shaped compact structure; translocation of nuclear pores; for the late phase: micronuclei formation and cytoplasm membrane disintegration).

This chapter describes an electron microscopy (EM) assay to detect apoptosis morphologically. An electron microscope is shown in **Fig. 2**. Cells are fixed, stained, dehydrated, embedded, cut into thin sections with an ultramicrotome (**Fig. 3**) and then cell sections are picked up on copper grids (**Fig. 4**). After poststaining, these sections can be viewed under an electron microscope. The steps leading up to and including the embedding step can be performed in a general laboratory. Subsequent steps require specialized equipment and training typically only found in an EM core facility.

2. Materials

2.1. Preparation of Cell Sections (see Note 1)

1. Phosphate-buffered saline (PBS): 37 mM NaCl, 2.7 mM KCl, 10 mM Na$_2$HPO$_4$, 1.4 mM KH$_2$PO$_4$, final pH 7.4. Stable at room temperature.

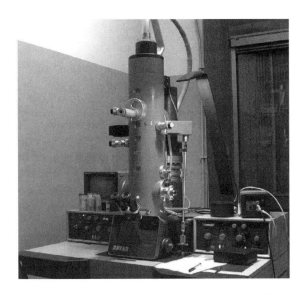

Fig. 2. Transmission electron microscope (TEM) ZEISS LEO EM 900.

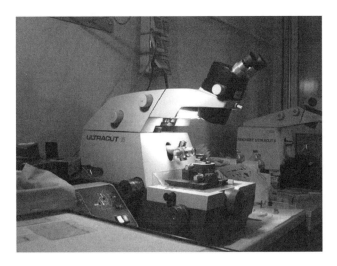

Fig. 3. PowerTome-XL ultramicrotome.

2. 0.25% (v/v) Trypsin, 1 mM ethylenediamine tetraacetic acid in PBS.
3. Fixing solution: 2% (v/v) glutaraldehyde (electron microscopy [EM] grade; *see* **Note 2**), 1% (w/v) tannic acid (EM grade; *see* **Note 2**) in 0.1 M sodium cacodylate (EM grade) pH 7.4.
4. Rinse solution: 0.1 M sodium cacodylate (EM grade), pH 7.4.

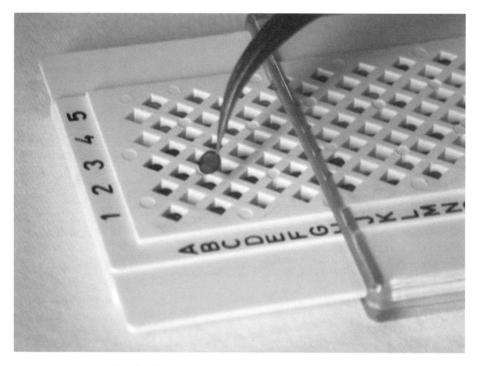

Fig. 4. Copper electron microscopy grids in box.

5. Osmium tetroxide (OsO_4) stain: 2% (w/v) osmium tetroxide in 0.1 M sodium cacodylate (EM grade), pH 7.4 (*see* **Note 3**).
6. 1% (w/v) Uranyl acetate in deionized H_2O (dH_2O; *see* **Note 4**).
7. 3% (w/v) Agarose (ultra-low gelling temperature, e.g., Sigma A-5030; *see* **Note 5**).
8. Acetone (EM grade).
9. Spurr's medium: 10 g vinylcyclohexene dioxide, 6 g diglycidyl ether of polypropyleneglycol (DER 736), 26 g nonenyl succinic anhydride, and 0.4 g dimethylaminoethanol (*see* **Note 6**).
10. Silicone mold (*see* **Note 7**).
11. Ultramicrotome.
12. Copper EM grid.
13. Bismuth subnitrate solution (50×): 2 M NaOH, add 0.17 M sodium tartrate dihydrate (EM grade), dissolve, 0.07 M bismuth subnitrate (EM grade). Store at 4°C for up to 2 wk (*see* **Note 8**).

3. Methods

3.1. Preparation of Cell Sections (see Note 9)

1. Detach about 10 million cells with trypsin. Pellet by centrifugation (400g, 5 min). Wash with ice-cold PBS. The cell pellet should be in the range of 1 mm^3.

2. Resuspend cells in 10 mL of the 2% glutaraldehyde fixing solution.
3. Fix cells by incubating overnight at 4°C.
4. Rinse the cells three times with the sodium cacodylate wash solution.
5. Resuspend the fixed cells in 3 mL of the OsO_4 stain solution. Allow staining for 1 to 2 h at room temperature with the tube wrapped with aluminum foil to prevent light mediated oxidation of the OsO_4.
6. Wash the cells three times with dH_2O.
7. Resuspend the cells in the 1% uranyl acetate. Allow staining for 15 min at room temperature.
8. Wash the cells three times with dH_2O.
9. Dissolve the agarose in dH_2O while being heated and allow cooling to 45°C. Resuspend the cells in the agarose by stirring with a spatula.
10. Pellet cells at 1000g for 10 min.
11. Allow the agarose to set at room temperature and then carefully cut off the bottom of the tube with a razor blade to obtain the pellet.
12. Transfer the cell pellet to a scintillation vial for the dehydration step, which involves incubating the pellet with increasing concentrations of acetone as follows, being certain that the cap is securely on at all times except during acetone exchanges. Start with 25% (v/v) acetone at room temperature, and every 10 min pour out the acetone and replace it with a higher concentration (i.e., 50%, 75%, 95%, 100%, 100%, and 100%).
13. Infiltrate the dehydrated cell pellet in Spurr's medium by incubating with increasing amounts of Spurr's medium as follows (*see* **Subheading 3.1.**, **steps 14–17**). The scintillation vial should be rotated during this process with the lid tightly screwed down except for medium exchanges.
14. Infiltrate for 1 h or more in one-third Spurr's medium and, two-thirds 100% acetone, at room temperature.
15. Remove the above mixture and replace with half Spurr's medium and half 100% acetone for 1 h or longer at room temperature.
16. Remove the above mixture and replace with two-thirds Spurr's medium and one-third 100% acetone for 1 h or longer at room temperature.
17. Remove the above mixture and replace with 100% Spurr's medium for not longer then 1 h at room temperature.
18. Place the pellet in a silicone mold filled with 100% Spurr's medium (*see* **Note 7**).
19. Polymerize in a convection oven for 65°C overnight.
20. The embedded cell pellet is now ready to cut. From now on, specialized facilities and training are required. Thin section the embedded pellet into 80-nm (gold) sections with an ultramicrotome.
21. Pick up the sections on a copper EM grid.
22. Poststain with 1% (w/v) uranyl acetate in dH_2O by floating the grid upside down on a 50-µL droplet of the solution on a sheet of parafilm (3–10 min, room temperature).
23. To remove the excess of uranyl acetate, wash the grid three to five times by rinsing on 50-µL droplets of filtered dH_2O for 1 min each.
24. Stain grid with the bismuth subnitrate solution for 3 to 10 min, at room temperature.

25. Rinse grid three times for 1 min each with filtered dH_2O.
26. Let grid dry at room temperature.
27. Observe grids in an EM.
28. Record micrographs on film, for example, Kodak 4489-sheet film or digitally if that option is available.

4. Notes

1. All reagents must be EM grade (e.g., from Polysciences, Warrington, PA) and filtered through a 0.22 µm filter prior to use. Any contamination by particulate matter will degrade the quality of the EM.
2. Use glutaraldehyde from a freshly opened ampoule of EM grade. Glutaraldehyde is the primary fixative and tannic acid is a mordant that facilitates binding of the osmium tetroxide to the fixed sample. Fresh vials of glutaraldehyde must be stored at 4°C in the dark and should appear clear. Do not use if it appears yellow.
3. Fresh vials of OsO_4 must be stored at 4°C in the dark and should appear pale yellow. Do not use if it appears gray or black. OsO_4 is an electron dense reagent that allows for lipid preservation and contrast for cell membranes under the EM.
4. The solution of Uranyl acetate must be made up, filtered and used on the same day. For the waste disposal, investigators must refer to the guidelines provided by their institutions.
5. The agarose serves to "glue" the cells together for the embedding procedure.
6. Spurr's medium is a resin designed for embedding for EM. It must be freshly prepared. Add the DMAE last after mixing the other components. These components are to be mixed in an airtight container such as a centrifuge tube, as they are highly hydroscopic and moisture in the mixture will prevent them from successfully polymerizing. Spurr's medium components can be obtained from companies that specialize in EM supplies (e.g., from Polysciences, Warrington, PA).
7. Silicone mold is just a container made of silicone. Inside the silicone mold there are many little wells, in which we pour the polymerizing resin. The wells contain alphanumeric self-impression cavities, which allow for the removal of the resin blocks after polymerization (Polysciences, Warrington, PA and Pelco International, Redding, CA). Silicone mold can be reused several times.
8. Bismuth subnitrate 50× solution is usually prepared in 10 mL of dH_2O. Begin by dissolving 8 g of NaOH and then dissolve 400 mg of sodium tartrate dihydrate. After this, add and dissolve 200 mg of bismuth subnitrate. To make working solution, dilute 20 µL of stock to 1 mL with dH_2O and filter.
9. All steps up to and including embedding in agarose must be done in a plastic 15-mL centrifuge tube and a benchtop centrifuge.

References

1. Tatton, W. G., Chalmers-Redman, R., Brown, D., and Tatton, N. (2003) Apoptosis in Parkinson's disease: signals for neuronal degradation. *Ann. Neurol.* **53(3 Suppl 1),** S61–S72.

2. Hickey, M. A. and Chesselet, M. F. (2003) Apoptosis in Huntington's disease. *Prog. Neuropsychopharmacol. Biol. Psychiatry* **27,** 255–265.

3. Mattson, M. P. (2002) Contributions of mitochondrial alterations, resulting from bad genes and a hostile environment, to the pathogenesis of Alzheimer's disease. *Int. Rev. Neurobiol.* **53,** 387–409.

4. Sabri, F., Titanji, K., De Milito, A., and Chiodi, F. (2003) Astrocyte activation and apoptosis: their roles in the neuropathology of HIV infection. *Brain Pathol.* **13,** 84–94.

5. Hildeman, D. A., Mitchell, T., Kappler, J., and Marrack, P. (2003) T cell apoptosis and rwactive oxygen species. *J. Clin. Invest.* **111,** 575–581.

6. El-Guendy, N. and Rangnekar, V. M. (2003) Apoptosis by Par-4 in cancer and neurodegenerative diseases. *Exp. Cell Res.* **283,** 51–66.

7. Shivapurkar, N., Reddy, J., Chaudhary, P. M., and Gazdar, A. F. (2003) Apoptosis and lung cancer: a review. *J. Cell. Biochem.* **88,** 885–898.

8. Hussein, M. R., Haemel, A. K., and Wood, G. S. (2003) Apoptosis and melanoma: molecular mechanisms. *J. Pathol.* **199,** 275–288.

9. Loro, L. L., Vintermyr, O. K., and Johannessen, A. C. (2003) Cell death regulation in oral squamous cell carcinoma: methodological considerations and clinical significance. *J. Oral Pathol. Med.* **32,** 125–138.

10. Coultas, L. and Strasser, A. (2003) The role of the Bcl-2 protein family in cancer. *Semin. Cancer Biol.* **13,** 115–123.

11. Kerr, J. F. R., Wyllie, A. H., and Currie, A. R. (1972) Apoptosis, a basic biological phenomenon with wide-ranging implications in tissue kinetics. *Br. J. Cancer* **26,** 239–257.

14

Detection of Apoptotic Deoxyribonucleic Acid Break by *In Situ* Nick Translation

Carmela Trimarchi, Dario La Sala, Alessandra Zamparelli, and Caterina Cinti

1. Introduction

Apoptosis plays a critical role in important biological processes such as morphogenesis, tissue homeostasis, and elimination of genomic damaged or virally infected cells and of self-reactive clones from the immune system (*1*). Although apoptosis is important during normal development, its aberrant activation may contribute to a number of diseases, such as AIDS, neurodegenerative disorders, and ischemic injury (*2*). However, impaired apoptosis may be a significant factor in the etiology of diseases like cancer, autoimmune disorders, and viral infections (*2*).

Cells can self-destruct via an intrinsic program of cell death (*1*). Morphologically, apoptosis is characterized by a series of structural changes in dying cells: blebbing of the plasma membrane, condensation of the cytoplasm and nucleus, and cellular fragmentation into membrane apoptotic bodies (*1,3*). Specifically, the cytoplasm begins to shrink after the cleavage of lamins and actin filaments. Nuclear condensation can also be observed after the breakdown of nuclear structural proteins, as well as chromatin progressive margination and compacting, with the final appearance of numerous and homogeneously dense micronuclei scattered throughout the cytoplasm (*3–5*). Cells continue to shrink, packaging themselves into a form that allows for easy clearance by macrophages. These phagocytic cells are responsible for removing apoptotic cells from tissues in a clean and tidy fashion that avoids many of the problems associated with necrotic cell death. Cells die in response to a variety of stimuli and during apoptosis they do so in a controlled, regulated fashion.

From: *Methods in Molecular Biology, Vol. 285: Cell Cycle Control and Dysregulation Protocols*
Edited by: A. Giordano and G. Romano © Humana Press Inc., Totowa, NJ

Biochemically, apoptosis is mostly correlated to the activation of Ca^{2+}/Mg^{2+}-dependent endonucleases, which determine blunt ended or double stranded deoxyribonucleic acid (DNA) breaks. This nicked DNA is subsequently cleaved in nucleosomic or oligonucleosomic fragments *(6–8)*. Initially, the chromatin is degraded into large fragments of 50–330 kilobases and subsequently into smaller fragments that are monomers and multimers of 200 base pairs *(3,9)*. Some studies demonstrated a correlation between DNA fragmentation and chromatin condensation close by nuclear lamina and, later, inside the micronuclei *(10)*.

Among the multiple technical approaches used for the study of apoptosis, the *in situ* nick translation (NT) represent a sensible method able to identify the presence of DNA breaks induced by Ca^{2+}/Mg^{2+}-dependent endonucleases. This technique is based on the ability of *Escherichia coli* DNA polymerase I enzyme (DNA Pol I) to bind both blunt ended and sticky ended nicked DNA. DNA Pol I synthesizes DNA complementary to the intact strand in a $5' \rightarrow 3'$ direction using the $3'$-OH termini of the nick as a primer. The $5' \rightarrow 3'$ exonucleolytic activity of DNA Pol I simultaneously removes nucleotides in the direction of the synthesis. The polymerase activity sequentially replaces nucleotides removed by exonucleolytic activity with new nucleotides reconstituting the intact DNA chain. The use of chemically labeled deoxyribonucleoside triphosphates (dNTPs) in the *in situ* NT reaction mixture and of fluorescein isothiocyanate (FITC)-conjugated antibody for the immunofluorescence detection allows to identify areas of green fluorescence corresponding to nicked DNA (**Fig. 1**).

This chapter describes the *in situ* NT technique to reveal the DNA breaks morphologically at early and late stages of apoptosis *(11)*. Cells are spread onto slides, fixed, and the DNA breaks of apoptotic cells are marked with digoxigenin-labeled dNTPs (DIG-dNTPs), revealed with anti-digoxygenin-fluorescein antibody (anti-DIG-FITC), and observed by confocal laser microscopy (**Fig. 2**).

2. Materials

1. 3:1 (v/v) Methanol/acetic acid solution (*see* **Note 1**).
2. Buffer I: 1 *M* Tris-HCl, 1 *M* NaCl, 0.04 *M* $MgCl_2$, 0.5% (v/v) Triton X-100, final pH 7.5 (*see* **Note 2**). Stable at room temperature.
3. Buffer II: 2% (w/v) bovine serum albumin in buffer I (*see* **Note 3**).
4. DNA polymerase I buffer: 500 m*M* TRIS-HCl (*see* **Note 4**), 50 m*M* $MgCl_2$, 100 m*M* 2-mercaptoethanole, final pH 7.8.
5. 1% (w/v) Trichloroacetic acid solution (TCA) in deionized H_2O (dH_2O; *see* **Note 5**).
6. DIG-DNA labeling mix: 1 m*M* dATP, 1 m*M* dCTP, 1 m*M* dGTP, 0.65 m*M* dTTP, and 0.35 m*M* digoxigenin-11-dUTP (DIG-11-UTP; *see* **Note 6**).
7. Reaction mix: 0.1 U/µL DNA polymerase I, 2% (v/v) DIG-DNA labeling mix, and 10% (v/v) DNA polymerase I buffer in sterile H_2O (*see* **Note 7**).

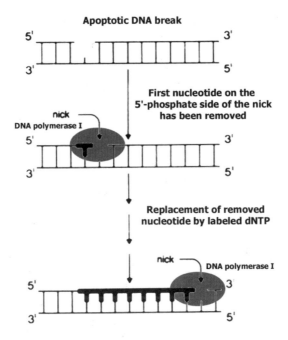

Fig. 1. Sequential action of DNA polymerase I (Pol I) during *in situ* NT reaction.

8. 200 µg/mL Anti-DIG-FITC (*see* **Note 8**).
9. Detection solution: 0.4 µg/mL anti-DIG-FITC, 10% (v/v) buffer II in deionized H₂O (dH₂O; *see* **Note 7**).
10. Phosphate-buffered saline (1×PBS): 37 mM NaCl, 2.7 mM KCl, 10 mM Na₂HPO₄, 1.4 mM KH₂PO₄, final pH 7.4. Stable at room temperature.
11. 1 µg/mL Propidium iodide (PI) in 1× PBS.
12. Permanent mounting medium.
13. Microscope glass slides.
14. Cover glass.
15. Thermostat water bath.
16. Orbital shaker.
17. Moist chamber.

3. Methods

3.1. Preparation of Slides

1. Detach about 5 million cells with trypsin. Transfer the cell suspension in a centrifuge tube. Pellet by centrifugation (400g, 10 min) and pipet off culture media. Wash the pellet in 1× PBS (*see* **Subheading 2.1.**, **step 10**).
2. After centrifugation remove the 1× PBS, maintain the tube with gently agitation (vortexing at low speed) and add, drop by drop, 1 mL of 3:1 (v/v) methanol:acetic

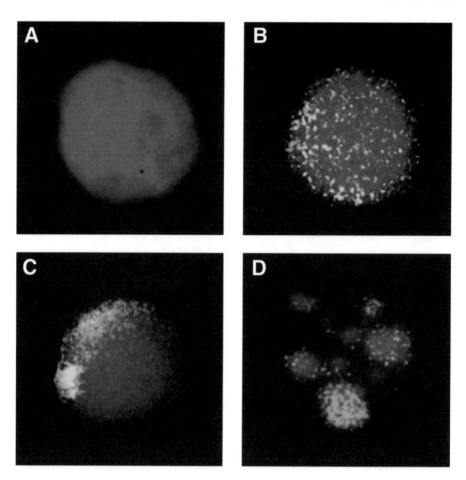

Fig. 2. Confocal laser microscopy images of nonapoptotic cell (**A**) and of *in situ* NT areas of cells in early (**B** and **C**) and late (**D**) apoptosis. The PI signal (in red) corresponds to areas of intact double-stranded DNA whereas the FITC signal (in green) shows the distribution of nicked DNA areas. At the early stages of apoptotic process the nicked DNA is initially homogeneously distributed in the whole nucleus (**B**), generating a spot-like pattern and subsequently is margined at the nuclear periphery appearing as cap-shaped compact structure (**C**). At the final apoptotic stage (late), the initial nuclear morphology is completely lost and the smaller fragments (monomers and multimers of 200 base pairs) of cleaved DNA are confined inside the micronuclei, which appear completely nicked (**D**). For the acquisition of images by confocal laser microscopy, FITC, and PI were excited with the blue (488 nm) and green (514 nm) line of the argon ion laser, respectively. Thereafter, serial optical sections of FITC signal, performed on *z*-axis and merged with the corresponding PI images, were elaborated and reconstructed as a three-dimensional projection.

acid (*see* **Subheading 2.1., step 1**) to fix cells. After the adding of fixing solution, stop the vortex and incubate the cells 30 min at room temperature.

3. Spread one to two drops of cell suspension onto slide and dry at room temperature until the complete evaporation of fixing solution.
4. Place slides in a slide rack and immerse 1 h in 1× PBS to rehydrate the cells (*see* **Subheading 2.1., step 10**).
5. Rinse the cells once in distilled H_2O and shake to wipe off excess of 1× PBS buffer.
6. Incubate each slide prepared with 50 µL of reaction mix at 37°C for 1 h in a moist chamber (*see* **Note 9**).
7. Put slides 5 min in the TCA solution at 4°C to remove the unincorporated dNTPs. Do not shake.
8. Rinse the slides 2 min in buffer I at room temperature.
9. Incubate the slides 20 min in buffer II at 42°C to stop the reaction. Do not shake.
10. Wash the slides twice in buffer I, 5 min/wash.
11. Keep slides in the dark in a slide box.
12. Lay the detection solution over spread cells and incubate 1 h in a moist chamber at 37°C in the dark (*see* **Note 9**).
13. Wash slides twice in buffer I at room temperature in the dark (5 min/wash).
14. Rinse slides twice in 1× PBS at room temperature in the dark (5 min/wash)
15. Incubate slides 4 mins with propidium iodide solution at room temperature in the dark.
16. Rinse slides twice in 1× PBS at room temperature in the dark (5 min/wash)
17. Dehydrate slides through alcohol as follows: 70% ethanol for 1 min, 95% ethanol for 1 min, and 100% ethanol for 1 min.
18. Wipe off excess ethanol and add one to two drops of permanent mounting medium and mount cover glass.
19. Observe slides by immunofluorescence or confocal laser microscopy.
20. Record digitally.

4. Notes

1. The solution must be precooled at –20°C prior to use.
2. TRIS powder must be completely dissolved in deionized H_2O, then adjust the pH to 7.5 with 37% HCl. Subsequently, add all the others components to complete the buffer (add Triton X-100 at the end of preparation).
3. The solution must be heated at 42°C in a water bath prior to use.
4. TRIS powder must be completely dissolved in deionized H_2O, then adjust the pH to 7.8 with 37% HCl; after the mix of all the buffer's components, the solution must be filtered through a 0.22-µm filter prior to use.
5. Trichloroacetic acid (TCA) is a hazardous compound; therefore, prepare the solution in a chemical hood. Trichloroacetic acid (TCA) is a hygroscopic powder and, therefore, do not use if it appears too hydrated. The solution must be stabilized on ice (4°C) prior to use.
6. All reagents are stable at –20°C. Repeated freezing and thawing should be avoided.
7. This solution must be freshly prepared prior to each use. Prepare 50 µL of mix for each slide.

8. The reconstituted solution is stable at –20°C. To avoid repeated freezing and thawing the solution must be stored in aliquot at –20°C protected from light.
9. 50 µL of reaction mix or detection solution should cover the area containing spread cells on each slide.

References

1. Steller H. (1995) Mechanisms and genes of cellular suicide (review). *Science* **267,** 1445–1449.
2. Thompson, C. B. (1995) Apoptosis in the pathogenesis and treatment of disease (review). *Science* **267,** 1456–1462.
3. Wyllie, A. H., Kerr, J. F. R., and Currie, A. R. (1980) Cell death: the significance of apoptosis. *Int. Rev. Cytol.* **68,** 251–306.
4. Arends, M. J. and Wyllie, A. H. (1991) Apoptosis: mechanisms and roles in pathology. *Int. Rev. Exp. Pathol.* **32,** 223–254.
5. Falcieri, E., Zamai, L., Santi, S., Cinti, C., Gobbi, P., Bosco, D., et al. (1994) The behaviour of nuclear domains in the course of apoptosis. *Histochemistry* **102,** 221–231.
6. Arends, M. J., Morris, R. G., and Wyllie, A. H. (1990) Apoptosis: the role of the endonuclease. *Am. J. Pathol.* **136,** 593–608.
7. Peitsch, C., Muller, C., and Tschopp, J. (1993) DNA fragmentation during apoptosis is caused by frequent single strand cuts. *Nucl. Acid Res.* **21,** 4206–4209.
8. Peitsch, M. C., Polzar, B., Stephan, H., Crompton, T., MacDonald, H. R., and Mannhertz, H. G. (1993) Characterization of the endogenous deoxyribonuclease involved in nuclear DNA degradation during apoptosis (programmed cell death). *EMBO J.* **12,** 371–377.
9. Oberhammer, F., Wilson, J. W., Dive, C., Morris, I. D., Hickman, J. A., Wakeling, A. E., et al. (1993) Apoptotic death in epithelial cells: cleavage of DNA to 300 and/or 50 Kb fragments prior or in absence of internucleosomal fragmentation. *EMBO J.* **12,** 3679–3684.
10. Falcieri, E., Suppia, L., Di Baldassarre, A., Mariani, A. R., Cinti, C., Columbaro, M., et al. (1996) Different approaches to the study of apoptosis. *Scan Microsc.* **10,** 227–237.
11. Lucchetti, F., Mariani, A. R., Columbaro, M., Di Baldassarre, A., Cinti, C., and Falcieri, E. (1998) Apoptotic pathways depend on the target enzymatic activity and not on the triggering agent. *Scanning* **21,** 29–35.

III

CELLULAR RESPONSE TO DEOXYRIBONUCLEIC ACID DAMAGE

15

Induction of Deoxyribonucleic Acid Damage by Alkylating Agents

Salvatore Cortellino, David P. Turner, Domenico Albino, and Alfonso Bellacosa

1. Introduction

Alkylating agents are a series of potentially carcinogenic compounds that are able to introduce lesions into deoxyribonucleic acid (DNA; **ref. 1**). For their electrophilic nature, alkylating agents have an affinity for the nucleophilic centers of DNA and are monofunctional (have one reactive group) or bifunctional (have two reactive groups). Alkylating agents, such as methylmethane-sulphonate and N-ethyl-N-nitrosourea, introduce methyl, ethyl, and complicated alkyl groups to the functional groups of nucleic acid bases, with ring nitrogens being generally more reactive than ring oxygens (*2–4*). The alkylation of oxygen in phosphodiester bonds results in phosphotriester formation (*5*) and bifunctional agents often react with two nucleophilic centers, producing inter- and intrastrand crosslinks (*6*).

Although the most frequent alkylated base is N'-alkylguanine, of particular biological importance is the generation of the alkylating product O^6-methyl-guanine, which base pairs with cytosine and thymine. Failure to repair this highly promutagenic lesion results in G:C to A:T transition mutations (*6*).

To protect genetic stability and the informational integrity of DNA, cells are armed with a series of DNA repair systems able to counteract the effects of alkylation (*6–8*). Repair failure results in damage accumulation, which triggers the cell to undergo cell cycle arrest and ultimately cell death through apoptosis. The same DNA repair systems that augment the repair of alkylation damage are also involved in cell cycle signaling (*9–11*).

From: *Methods in Molecular Biology, Vol. 285: Cell Cycle Control and Dysregulation Protocols*
Edited by: A. Giordano and G. Romano © Humana Press Inc., Totowa, NJ

Alkylating agents are used as chemotherapeutic agents in the fight against cancer and have important applications in the laboratory *(12)*. Exposing cells to these agents allows a mechanistic study into DNA repair, cell cycle signaling, and apoptosis. *N*-methyl-*N'*-nitrosoguanidine (MNNG) is an example of an alkylating agent that in vivo becomes a highly reactive methylating agent. In this chapter, we describe how to treat cells with MNNG and how to process them for 3-(4,5-dimethylthiazol-2-yl)-2,5-diphenyl tetrazolium bromide (MTT) assay. This is a colorimetric assay that measures the reduction of MTT by mitochondrial succinate dehydrogenase. Because the reduction of MTT can only occur in metabolically active cells, the level of activity is a measure of the cell viability.

2. Materials

2.1. Routine Cell Culture

1. Dulbecco's Modified Eagle Medium (DMEM) supplemented with 15% fetal calf serum, 1 mM sodium pyruvate, 2 mM glutamine, 10 U/mL penicillin, and 10 µg/mL streptomycin (Gibco, Rockville, MD).
2. Falcon T-75 250 mL straight-necked flasks with a 0.2-µm vent (Fisher Scientific, Suwanne, GA).
3. Human diploid fibroblast wash buffer: 137 mM NaCl, 5 mM KCl, 4 mM NaHCO$_3$, 0.5 mM ethylenediamine tetraacetic acid, 0.1% (w/v) glucose, final pH 7.4 (Gibco, Rockville, MD).
4. 0.04% (v/v) Trypsin (Gibco, Rockville, MD).
5. 15-mL Falcon tubes (Fisher Scientific, Suwanne, GA).
6. Suitable microscope for visualizing cells.

2.2. MNNG Treatment

1. MNNG 10 mg/mL in DMSO (Sigma, 129941-10G).
2. *See* **Subheading 2.1.**, step 1.

2.3. Preparation of Cells for MTT Assay

1. Phosphate buffered saline: 37 mM NaCl, 2.7 mM KCl, 10 mM Na$_2$HPO$_4$, 1.4 mM KH$_2$PO$_4$, final pH 7.4. Stable at room temperature.
2. MTT (Sigma, M-2128). Prepare a 5 mg/mL solution in sterile phosphate-buffered saline, filter through 0.22-µm filter, and bring to 37°C before use. Make fresh at least each month. Store at 4°C in the dark.
3. Lysis buffer: 50% (v/v) *N,N*-dimethyl formamide, 2.5% (v/v) glacial acetic acid [the initial concentration is 80%(v/v)], 2.5% (v/v) HCl (the initial concentration is 1 N). Bring pH to 4.7. Add 20% (w/v) sodium dodecyl sulfate (SDS; *see* **Note 1**). Mix, heat, and filter sterilize. Store at room temperature. Bring to 37°C before use.
4. Multi channel pipet.
5. ELISA reader (Multiskan Ascent, ThermoLabsystems, Marietta, OH).

3. Methods

3.1. Routine Cell Culture (see Note 2)

1. Original mouse embryo fibroblasts are grown in DMEM and routinely divided when growth had reached 80–90% confluence. Typically, they are split one to three every 3 d.
2. Aspirate off the old media and wash the cells with 6 mL of human diploid fibroblast wash buffer before aspirating again.
3. Detach the cells from the flask by adding 3 mL of 0.04% (v/v) trypsin and incubate at 37°C in 5% CO_2 incubator for 5 min.
4. When the cells have detached from the flask (as monitored under a microscope) harvest the cells in 9 mL of DMEM and transfer into 15-mL Falcon tubes for cell counting.
5. Plate the cells in 96-well plate at a density of 4000 cells/well.

3.2. Treatment With MNNG

1. Remove the medium from the 96-well plate, aspirating from the wells with a Pasteur pipet connected to a vacuum system.
2. Pipet 100 µL of DMEM with different concentrations of MNNG (typical range between 0.3 to 10 µg/mL) in each well. Typically, all the wells in a column receive the same concentration of MNNG.
3. As a control, pipet 100 µL of DMEM + DMSO in all the wells of a few columns.
4. Incubate the plate at 37°C in 5% CO_2 and air, typically for 2–5 d.

A typical arrangement of a plate is shown in **Fig. 1**.

3.3. Preparation of Cells for MTT Assay

1. Add 25 µL of MTT solution to the wells. Leave a few wells in each column without MTT as additional control (**Fig. 1**). This will allow one to assess the background.
2. Incubate the plate for 2 h at 37°C in 5% CO_2 incubator.
3. Add 100 µL of lysis buffer to each well.
4. Incubate overnight at 37°C in 5% CO_2 incubator (typically 16 h).
5. Read the plate at 570 nm single wavelength with 5 s mixing.

3.4. Data Analysis

1. From the average OD the DMSO control column subtract average OD of the no MTT column (background).
2. From the average OD of each treatment column subtract average of the no MTT column (background).
3. Calculate percent survival as the ratio of the following:

$$\frac{\text{Background} - \text{subtracted average treatment OD}}{\text{Background} - \text{subtracted average DMSO control OD}} \times 100$$

4. Plot the data (average ± standard deviation) for each MNNG concentration.

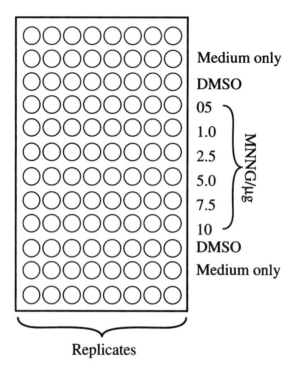

Medium only
DMSO
05 ⎫
1.0 ⎪
2.5 ⎬ MNNG/µg
5.0 ⎪
7.5 ⎪
10   ⎭
DMSO
Medium only

Replicates

Fig. 1. Arrangement of samples in a 96-well plate for MTT assay after MNNG treatment.

4. Notes

1. SDS may damage the electrode of the pH meter. Adjust the pH before adding SDS to the solution.
2. Mouse embryo fibroblasts are routinely grown in T-75 250 mL straight-necked flasks with a 0.2-µm vent at 37°C in 5% CO_2 incubator.

References

1. Lawley, P. D. (1989) Mutagens as carcinogens: development of current concept. *Mutat. Res.* **213,** 3–25.
2. Lawley, P. D. (1966) Effects of some chemical mutagens and carcinogens on nucleic acid. *Prog. Nucleic Acid Res. Mol. Biol.* **5,** 89–131.
3. Loveless, A. (1966) *Genetic and Allied Effects of Alkylating Agents.* Butterworths, London.
4. Roberts, J. J. (1978) The repair of DNA modified by cytotoxic, mutagenic, and carcinogenic chemicals. *Adv. Radiat. Biol.* **7,** 211–435.
5. Singer, B. (1986) O-Alkyl pyrimidines in mutagenesis and carcinogenesis: occurrence and significance. *Cancer Res.* **46,** 4879–4885

6. Friedberg, E. C., Walker, G. C., and Siede, W. (1995) *DNA Repair and Mutagenesis*. ASM Press, Washington.
7. Schendel, P. F. and P. E. Robins. (1978) Repair of O^6-methylguanine in adapted *Escherichia coli. Proc. Natl. Acad. Sci. USA* **75,** 6017–6020.
8. Boulden, A. M., Foote, R. S., Fleming, G. S., and Mitra, S. (1987) Purification and some properties of human O6-methylguanine methyltransferase. *J. Biosci.* **11,** 215–224.
9. Tronov V. A., Konstantinov E. M., and Kramarenko I. I. (2002) Role of excision mechanisms of DNA repair in induction of apoptosis. *Biochemistry (Mosc)* **67,** 730–736.
10. Bernstein C., Bernstein H., Payne C. M., and Garewal H. (2002) DNA repair/proapoptotic dual-role proteins in five major DNA repair pathways: fail-safe protection against carcinogenesis. *Mutat. Res.* **511,** 145–178.
11. Bellacosa, A. (2001) Functional interactions and signaling properties of mammalian DNA mismatch repair proteins. *Cell Death Differ.* **8,** 1076–1092.
12. Margison G. P., Santibanez Koref, M. F., and Povey A. C. (2002) Mechanisms of carcinogenicity/chemotherapy by O6-methylguanine. *Mutagenesis* **17,** 483–487.

16

Induction of Deoxyribonucleic Acid Damage by γ Irradiation

Salvatore Cortellino, David P. Turner, and Alfonso Bellacosa

1. Introduction

γ Radiation is an electromagnetic radiation with wavelengths in the range of 0.1–100 pm. Like all forms of electromagnetic radiations, the γ ray has no mass and no charge and interacts with material by colliding with the electrons in the shells of atoms. Irradiation with γ rays is very penetrating, and the energy transferred induces a wide variety of lesions into the components of cultured cells, especially deoxyribonucleic acid (DNA).

DNA damage is introduced in two ways. The first is through the direct ionization of DNA components and accounts for approx 35% of the cell killing caused by γ irradiation *(1,2)*. The remaining 65% is caused by the indirect ionization of H_2O, which greatly increases the concentration of reactive oxygen products within the cell *(1,2)*.

Radical species, such as primarily hydroxy radicals, but also hydrogen peroxide and peroxide radicals, react with DNA either directly or indirectly *(1)*. Radical attack causes base loss and single- and double-strand breaks and also generates several mutagenic DNA products, including thymine glycol, 8-hydroxyguanine; 4,6-diamino-5-formamidopyrimidine; and 2,6-diamino-4-hydroxy-5-formamidopyrimidine *(3–7)*.

Cell killing by γ radiation is described by the linear-quadratic model. This model separates cell killing into two components, α and β, corresponding to single-hit and double-hit kinetics of cell death, respectively *(8)*. α Inactivation represents most of cell killing with a 2-Gy fraction, whereas β inactivation becomes more important at doses >5-Gy *(8)*.

From: *Methods in Molecular Biology, Vol. 285: Cell Cycle Control and Dysregulation Protocols*
Edited by: A. Giordano and G. Romano © Humana Press Inc., Totowa, NJ

To preserve DNA stability and cell viability, cells are armed with a series of DNA repair systems able to counteract the effects of gamma irradiation *(3)*. However, when the damage is beyond the capabilities of the repair pathways, checkpoints are triggered, leading to cell cycle arrest and apoptosis *(9)*. γ Irradiation therefore has proved a useful tool in the study of the cell cycle and apoptosis through an examination of the responses caused by its exposure to cultured cells.

In this chapter, we will outline the γ irradiation of cells in preparation for apoptosis analysis using the Cell Death Detection Elisa^PLUS (Roche, Mannheim, Germany). This photometric immunoassay measures mono- and oligo-nucleosomes present in the cytoplasm induced after cell death.

2. Materials
2.1. Routine Cell Culture

1. Dulbecco's Modified Eagle Medium (DMEM) supplemented with 15% fetal calf serum, 1 mM sodium pyruvate, 2 mM glutamine, 10 U/mL penicillin, and 10 μg/mL streptomycin (Gibco, Rockville, MD).
2. Falcon T-75, 250-mL straight-necked flasks with a 0.2-μm vent (Fisher Scientific, Suwanne, GA).
3. Human diploid fibroblast wash buffer: 137 mM NaCl, 5 mM KCl, 4 mM NaHCO$_3$, 0.5 mM ethylenediamine tetraacetic acid (EDTA), 0.1% (w/v) glucose, final pH 7.4 (Gibco, Rockville, MD).
4. 0.04% (v/v) Trypsin (Gibco, Rockville, MD).
5. 15-mL Falcon tubes (Fisher Scientific, Suwanne, GA).
6. Suitable microscope for visualizing cells.

2.2. Cell Irradiation

1. DMEM supplemented with 15% fetal calf serum, 1 mM sodium pyruvate, 2 mM glutamine, 10 U/mL penicillin, and 10 μg/mL streptomycin (Gibco, Rockville, MD).
2. Falcon 60 × 15-mm tissue culture dishes (Fisher Scientific, Suwanne, GA).
3. Cesium-137 panoramic gamma irradiator Shepherd Model 81–14R, in a shielded experimental room (**Fig. 1**). This is a 6000 Ci irradiator that produces a vertical or horizontal beam of high intensity gamma rays. Dose rates of 10 Gy/min and less can be produced within fields of different sizes, depending on distance of the specimen from the radiation source.

2.3. Apoptosis Assay Cell Death Detection Elisa^PLUS

1. Phosphate-buffered saline (PBS): 37 mM NaCl, 2.7 mM KCl, 10 mM Na$_2$HPO$_4$, 1.4 mM KH$_2$PO$_4$, final pH 7.4. Stable at room temperature. It can be used with or without 0.1% (w/v) EDTA.
2. 15-mL Falcon tubes (Fisher Scientific, Suwanne, GA).
3. Cell scrapers (Fisher Scientific, Suwanne, GA).
4. Eppendorf tubes.

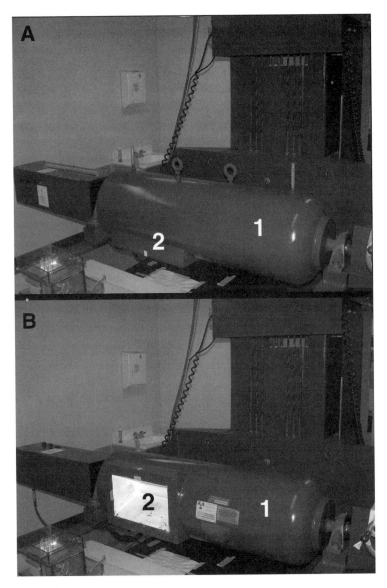

Fig. 1. The Cesium-137 panoramic γ irradiator Shepherd Model 81–14R. (**A**) The radioactive source is located in a lead-shielded cylindrical casing (1). During irradiation, the source is moved toward the irradiation port (2). (**B**) The cylindrical casing (1) is rotated 90° to improve the visualization of the irradiation port (2).

5. Rotating wheel (Labquake 415110, Barnstead/Thermolyne, Iowa).
6. Centrifuge (it must be able to hold 15-mL Falcon tubes).
7. Cell Death Detection Elisa^PLUS Lysis buffer (Roche, Mannheim, Germany).
8. Cell Death Detection Elisa^PLUS Immunoreagent prepared by mixing 1/20 volume anti-DNA-peroxidase and 1/20 volume anti-histone-biotin with 18/20 volumes of incubation buffer. These antibodies allow for the detection and quantification of mono- and oligonucleosomes that are present in the cytoplasmatic fraction of cell lysates. Mono- and oligonucleosomes are generated during apoptosis from cleavage of double-stranded DNA by endogenous endonuclease at internucleosomal linker region.
9. Cell Death Detection Elisa^PLUS ABTS substrate solution.
10. Cell Death Detection Elisa^PLUS Incubation buffer.
11. Multi Plates shaker.
12. ELISA reader (Multiskan Ascent, ThermoLabsystems, Marietta, OH).
13. Multi-channel pipet.

3. Methods

3.1. Routine Cell Culture (see Note 1)

1. Original mouse embryonic fibroblasts are grown in DMEM and routinely divided when growth had reached 80–90% confluence. Typically, they are split one to three every 3 d.
2. Aspirate off the old media and wash the cells with 6 mL of human diploid fibroblast wash buffer before aspirating again (*see* **Note 2**).
3. Detach the cells from the flask by adding 3 mL of 0.04% (v/v) trypsin and incubate for 5 min at 37°C in 5% CO_2 incubator.
4. When the cells have detached from the flask (as monitored under a microscope) harvest the cells in 9 mL of DMEM and transfer into 15-mL Falcon tubes for quantification.
5. Plate the cells in Falcon 60 × 15 mm tissue culture dish at a density of 7×10^4 cells/plate (approx 50% confluent). Incubate for 24 h at 37°C in 5% CO_2 incubator.

3.2. Cell Irradiation

1. Remove old medium from the culture dish and replace with fresh medium.
2. Place the plates with plastic lids under the γ-ray source and arrange in a symmetrical pattern.
3. Irradiate with different doses (typically 0.5–10 Gy).
4. Always include untreated control plates in the experiment (*see* **Note 3**).
5. After γ irradiation, incubate the plates for 3–5 d at 37°C in 5% CO_2 incubator (*see* **Note 4**).

3.3. Preparation of Cells for Apoptosis Assay

1. Collect the medium in 15-mL Falcon tubes.
2. Scrape the cells into 3 mL of PBS without EDTA.

3. Transfer PBS with scraped cells into the same 15-mL Falcon tubes, combining with medium from **Subheading 3.3., step 1**.

4. Pellet the cells at 500g for 10 min and discard the supernatant.

5. Resuspend the cell pellet with 70 μL of lysis buffer and transfer into Eppendorf tubes.

6. Incubate for 30 min at room temperature on a rotating wheel.

7. Centrifuge samples at 1800g for 10 min.

8. Transfer 20 μL of cell lysate supernatant into individual wells of streptavidin-coated multi plates (MTPs).

9. To a few fresh wells, add 20 μL of positive control for apoptosis (*see* **Note 5**).

10. Dispense 80 μL of the immunoreagent into each well.

11. Cover the MTP with adhesive cover foil, place on shaker and gently shake for 2 h at room temperature.

12. Remove the solution by suction and rinse the wells three times with 200 μL of incubation buffer.

13. Add 100 μL of ABTS solution to each well.

14. Incubate on MTP shaker until color development is sufficient for photometric analysis.

15. Measure OD at 405 nm and 490 nm for each well (*see* **Note 6**).

3.4. Data Analysis

1. Subtract the background value of the immunoassay (OD_{490}) from the specific signal (OD_{405}).

2. Calculate the specific enrichment of mono- and oligonucleosomes released into cytoplasm using the following formula:

$$\frac{\text{Background} - \text{subtracted absorbance of the sample}}{\text{Background} - \text{subtracted absorbance of untreated control cells}}$$

3. Plot the relative enrichment as a function of radiation dose.

4. Notes

1. Mouse embryo fibroblasts are routinely grown in T-75, 250-mL straight-necked flasks with a 0.2-μm vent at 37°C in 5% CO_2 incubator.

2. Apoptotic or dying cells may have detached from the plastic and may be present in the medium.

3. Untreated control plates are left outside the shielded irradiation room for the entire irradiation time.

4. In an alternative protocol, the cell culture is trypsinized and the cell suspension is transferred into medium supplemented with serum. While the cells' suspension is slowly stirred, the radiation dose is delivered. A portion of irradiated cells is removed and placed on ice to minimize DNA repair. The next radiation dose is delivered to the remainder of the cell suspension. After each dose fraction, a portion of irradiated cells is removed, as described in **Subheading 3.2., steps 1–5**.

5. The positive control is DNA–histone complex stabilized.
6. Absorbance at 405 nm represents specific antibody signal. Absorbance at 490 nm represents background from the ABTS solution.

References

1. Goodhead, D. T. (1989) The initial damage produced by ionizing radiations. *Int. J. Radiat. Biol.* **56,** 623–634.
2. Ward, J. F. (1988) DNA damage produced by ionizing radiation in mammalian cells: identities, mechanisms of formation and reparability. *Prog. Nucleic Acid Res. Mol. Biol.* **35,** 95–125.
3. Friedberg, E. C., Walker, G. C., and Siede, W. (1995) *DNA Repair and Mutagenesis*, ASM Press, Washington.
4. Riley, P. A. (1994) Free radicals in biology: oxidative stress and the effects of ionizing radiation. *Int. J. Radiat. Biol.* **65,** 27–33.
5. Cerruti, P. A. (1976) DNA base damage induced by ionizing radiation, in *Photochemestry and Pothobiology of Nucleic Acids* (Wang, S. Y., ed.), Academic Press, Inc., New York, p. 375–401
6. Ward, J. F. (1990) The yield of DNA double-strand breaks produced intracellularly by ionizing radiation: a review. *Int. J. Radiat. Biol.* **57,** 1141–1150.
7. Olive, P. G. (1998) The role of DNA single- and double-strand breaks in cell killing by ionizing radiation. *Radiat. Res.* **150(Suppl),** S42–S51.
8. Chapman, J. D., Stobbe, C. C., Gales, T., Das, I. J., Zellmer, D. L., Biade, S., et al. (1999) Condensed chromatin and cell inactivation by single-hit kinetics. *Radiat. Res.* **151,** 433–441.
9. Bellacosa, A. (2001) Functional interactions and signaling properties of mammalian DNA mismatch repair proteins. *Cell Death Differ.* **8,** 1076–1092.

17

Ultraviolet Irradiation of Cells

David P. Turner, Anthony T. Yeung, and Alfonso Bellacosa

1. Introduction

Ultraviolet (UV) radiation is mutagenic in a wide variety of organisms and is a major source of physical deoxyribonucleic acid (DNA) damage. The mutations caused and the biological consequences of exposing cell cultures to UV light have been extensively studied and have given many insights into the underlying mechanisms that lie behind DNA damage and repair *(1–3)*. UV radiation occurs at three wavelengths: 400 to 320 nm (UV-A), 320 to 290 nm (UV-B), and 290 to 100 nm (UV-C). Although UV-C is generally accepted to be the most harmful source of UV radiation, it occurs mainly in artificial light, as opposed to UV-A and B, which occur naturally in the environment as solar radiation.

The main mutagenic lesions caused by UV irradiation are cyclobutane pyrimidine dimers and pyrimidine-pyrimidone 6–4 photoproducts (6-4PPs; **refs. *3–5***). Less common products include thymine glycols and double strand breaks *(3)*. All of these lesions have been shown to block transcription in vivo and in vitro *(6,7)* and have been implicated in signaling cell cycle arrest and apoptosis *(8)*. UV irradiation therefore has proved to be a useful tool in the examination of cell cycle checkpoints through an examination of the responses caused by its exposure to cultured cells *(9–11)*. In this chapter, we will outline the UV irradiation of cells in preparation for cell cycle analysis by fluorescence-activated cell sorting (FACS) and protein analysis by Western blotting.

2. Materials

2.1. Routine Cell Culture

1. Dulbecco's Modified Eagle Medium (DMEM) supplemented with 15% fetal calf serum, 1 m*M* sodium pyruvate, 2 m*M* glutamine, 10 U/mL penicillin, and 10 µg/mL streptomycin (Gibco, Rockville, MD).

From: *Methods in Molecular Biology, Vol. 285: Cell Cycle Control and Dysregulation Protocols*
Edited by: A. Giordano and G. Romano © Humana Press Inc., Totowa, NJ

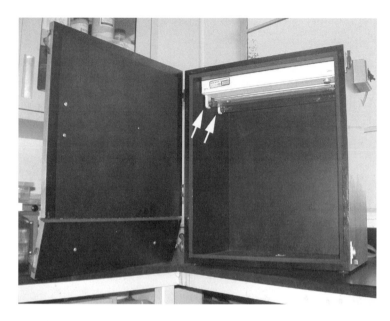

Fig. 1. Typical set up for UV irradiation. The arrows depict the germicidal lamps, which are located in a dark box. Cell culture plates will be placed on a surface for UV irradiation approx 45 cm away from the germicidal lamps.

2. Falcon T-75 250-mL straight-necked flasks with a 0.2-μm vent (Fisher Scientific, Suwanne, GA).
3. Human diploid fibroblast (HDF) wash buffer: 137 mM NaCl, 5 mM KCl, 4 mM NaHCO$_3$, 0.5 mM ethylenediamine tetraacetic acid (EDTA), 0.1% (w/v) glucose, final pH 7.4 (Gibco, Rockville, MD).
4. 0.04% Trypsin (Gibco, Rockville, MD).
5. 15-mL Falcon tubes (Fisher Scientific, Suwanne, GA).
6. Suitable microscope for visualizing cells.

2.2. Cell Irradiation

1. *See* **Subheading 2.1.**, **step 3**.
2. 15 watt, 17 inches long, GE germicidal lamp (no. G15T8; **Fig. 1**).

2.3. Preparation of Cells for FACS

1. Phosphate buffered saline (PBS): 37 mM NaCl, 2.7 mM KCl, 10 mM Na$_2$HPO$_4$, 1.4 mM KH$_2$PO$_4$, final pH 7.4. Stable at room temperature. It may supplied with or without 0.1% EDTA.
2. 15-mL Falcon tubes (Fisher Scientific, Suwanne, GA).

3. Centrifuge (it must be able to hold 15-mL Falcon tubes).
4. 70% Ethanol.
5. Vortex.
6. Fetal calf serum (*see* **Note 1**).
7. Propidium iodide (20 µg/mL)/Rnase A (250 µg/mL) solution in PBS without EDTA, supplemented with 1% fetal calf serum (*see* **Note 2**).

2.4. Protein Extraction

1. Dulbecco's PBS containing Ca^{2+} and Mg^{2+} (Gibco, Rockville, MD).
2. RIPA buffer; 50 mM Tris-HCl, pH 7.5; 150 mM NaCl; 1% (v/v) Triton X-100; 0.5% (v/v) sodium deoxycholate; 0.1 M sodium fluoride; 0.1% (w/v) SDS, filter sterilize. Add inhibitors immediately before use to the following final concentrations: 100 mM sodium orthovanadate, 100 mM sodium pyrophosphate, 1 mM phenylmethyl sulfonyl fluoride, 1 mM dithiothreitol, 1 mM EDTA, 10 µg/mL aprotinin and 10 µg/mL leupeptin (*see* **Note 3**).
3. Cell scraper (Gibco, Rockville, MD).
4. 15-mL Falcon tubes (Fisher Scientific, Suwanne, GA).
5. *See* **Subheading 2.3., step 3**.
6. Sonication equipment.
7. Microcentrifuge.
8. Liquid nitrogen.

3. Methods
3.1. Routine Cell Culture (see Note 4)

1. Original mouse embryo fibroblast stocks are grown in DMEM media and routinely divided when growth had reached 80–90% confluence. Typically, they are split one to three every 3 d.
2. Aspirate off the old media and wash the cells with 6 mL of HDF wash buffer before aspirating again.
3. Detach the cells from the flask by adding 3 mL of 0.04% (v/v) trypsin and incubate at 37°C in 5% CO_2 incubator for 5 min.
4. When the cells have detached from the flask (as monitored under a microscope) harvest the cells in 9 mL of DMEM media and transfer into 15-mL Falcon tubes for cell counting (*see* **Note 5**).

3.2. Cell Irradiation

1. Remove and retain the medium from the culture flasks.
2. Wash the MEF twice with HDF buffer, aspirating the buffer away each time.
3. Place the plates uncovered under the UV lamp and irradiate at a distance of 45 cm from the cells at a dosage of 2 J/m²/s (*see* **Note 6**).
4. After UV irradiation, replace the original retained media and further incubate for 30 min at 37°C in 5% CO_2 incubator.

3.3. Preparation of Cells for FACS

1. Harvest the MEF cells by trypsinization as outlined in **Subheading 3.1., steps 1–4**.
2. Pellet the cells at 500g for 5 min and discard the supernatant.
3. Wash the pellet with PBS without EDTA.
4. Discard the supernatant and re-suspend pellet in 0.5 mL of PBS without EDTA.
5. While gently vortexing the cells, add 5 mL of 70% ethanol in order to fix the cells for analysis (*see* **Note 7**).
6. Leave the cells in fixative for at least 15 min at 4°C (*see* **Note 8**).
7. Centrifuge at 500g for 5 min and wash with 5 mL of PBS supplemented with 1% fetal calf serum.
8. Discard the supernatant and re-suspend the pellet in 300 µL of propidium iodide/RNase A solution (*see* **Note 2**) and incubate for 30 min at 37°C.
9. Analyze the cells within 24 h. Store the cells in the propidium iodide/RNase A solution protected from light at 4°C.

3.4. Protein Extraction

1. Wash the MEF with 5 mL of Dulbecco's PBS containing Ca^{2+} and Mg^{2+}.
2. Aspirate the wash, add a further 5 mL of PBS and detach the adherent cells using a sterile cell scraper.
3. Transfer the detached cells into 10-mL Falcon tubes and pellet at 200g for 5 min.
4. Discard supernatant, then on ice, add 100 µL of lysis buffer and transfer the cells to prechilled Eppendorf tubes and incubate on ice for 15 min.
5. Keeping the cells on ice, sonicate at 60 Hz for 30 s. Repeat the sonication four times with a 1-min interval between each sonication step.
6. Transfer the lysate to fresh Eppendorf tubes and spin at maximum speed for 10 min at 4°C.
7. Transfer the supernatant containing the protein lysate, into fresh tubes and calculate the protein concentration (*see* **Note 9**).
8. If storage is required, freeze in liquid nitrogen and store at –80°C.

4. Notes

1. The supplemented serum may vary, as different cell lines require different types and levels of nutrients. For example, MEF cells are best cultured in fetal calf serum, while NIH 3T3 cells growth better in calf serum.
2. It is best to make this fresh from stock solutions before use. Propidium iodide is a nucleic acid fluorescent stain. The membrane permeability of propidium iodide varies between live, dead and apoptotic cells. The addition of Rnase A is required to remove RNA before analysis.
3. It is important that the inhibitors are added immediately before use as they degrade quickly.
4. Mouse embryo fibroblasts are routinely grown in T-75 250-mL straight-necked flasks with a 0.2-µm vent at 37°C in 5% CO_2 incubator. All work conducted with MEF cells should be performed in Class II cabinets using aseptic technique at all times. All media and reagents should be pre-warmed before use.

5. Cell counting is commonly performed manually using a hemocytometer chamber counter (Fisher Scientific, Suwanne, GA) or mechanically using a cell counter, such as a Coulter Counter (Beckman Coulter, Fullerton, CA).
6. The extent to which UV irradiation initiates DNA lesions is cell-, wavelength-, dose-, and time-dependent. The literature states that exposure to 1 J/m^2 does not greatly effect colony formation efficiency. Doses between 5 and 10 J/m^2 reduce colony formation by 50 to 70% and doses of >40 J/m^2 reduce efficiency by <95% *(9)*.
7. It is important that the cells do not clump together and this can be avoided by gentle slow vortexing.
8. Fixed cells can be stored in this manner for several weeks.
9. The protein concentration in the cell lysate can be calculated using the Bio-Rad protein assay kit (Bio-Rad Laboratories, Hercules, CA).

References

1. Moan, J. and Peak, M. J. (1989) Effects of UV radiation of cells. *J. Photochem. Photobiol.* **4,** 21–34.
2. Tornaletti, S. and Pfeifer, G. P. (1996) UV damage and repair mechanisms in mammalian cells. *Bioessays* **18,** 221–228.
3. Friedberg, E. C., Walker, G. C., and Siede, W. (1995) *DNA Repair and Mutagenesis*, ASM Press, Washington.
4. Yoon, J-H., Lee, C-S., O'Conner, T. R., Yasui, A., and Pfeifer, G. P. (2000) The DNA damage spectrum produced by simulated sunlight. *J. Mol. Biol.* **299,** 681–693.
5. Varghese, A. J. (1972) Photochemistry of nucleic acids and their constituents. *Photophysiology* **7,** 207–274.
6. Donahue, B. A., Yin, S., Taylor, J. S., Reines, D., and Hanawalt, P. C. (1994) Transcript cleavage by RNA polymerase II arrested by a cyclobutane pyrimidine dimer in the DNA template. *Proc. Natl. Acad. Sci. USA* **91,** 8502–8506.
7. van Hoffen, A., Venema, J., Meschini, R., van Zeeland, A. A., and Mullenders, L. H. (1995) Transcription-coupled repair removes both cyclobutane pyrimidine dimers and 6–4 photoproducts with equal efficiency and in a sequential way from transcribed DNA in xeroderma pigmentosum group C fibroblasts. *EMBO J.* **14,** 360–367.
8. Bill, C. A. and Nickoloff, J. A. (2000) Ultraviolet light induced and spontaneous recombination in eukaryotes, in *DNA Damage and Repair, Vol 3: Advances from Phage to Humans* (Nickoloff, J. A. and Hoekstra, M. F., eds.), Humana Press, Totowa, NJ pp. 329–357.
9. Heffernan, T. P., Simpson, D. A., Frank, A. R., Heinloth, A. N., Paules, R. S., Cordeiro-Stone, M., et al. (2002) An ATR- and Chk1-dependent S checkpoint inhibits replicon initiation following UVC induced DNA damage. *Mol. Cell Biol.* **22,** 8552–8561.
10. Wright, J. A., Keegan, K. S., Herendeen, D. R., Bently, N. J., Carr, A. M., Hoekstra, M. F., et al. (1998) Protein kinases mutants of human ATR increase sensitivity to UV and ionizing radiation and abrogate cell cycle checkpoint control. *Proc. Natl. Acad. Sci. USA* **95,** 7445–7450.
11. Sanchez, Y. and Elledge, S. J. (1995) Stopped for repairs. *Bioessays* **17,** 545–548.

IV

RETROVIRIDAE-BASED VECTORS: PROTOCOLS FOR LENTIVIRAL- AND RETROVIRAL-MEDIATED GENE TRANSFER TO ENGINEER CELL CULTURE SYSTEMS

18

Transient Production of Retroviral- and Lentiviral-Based Vectors for the Transduction of Mammalian Cells

Tiziana Tonini, Pier Paolo Claudio, Antonio Giordano, and Gaetano Romano

1. Introduction

The genera of the retroviridae comprise oncoretroviruses and lentiviruses *(1)*. Oncoretroviruses can only infect dividing cells, as they require the breakdown of the nuclear membrane to access the cellular chromosomal deoxyribonucleic acid (DNA; **ref. 2**). Conversely, lentiviruses can also infect nondividing cells *(3)*. Retroviral and lentiviral vectors are among the most powerful techniques for gene delivery into mammalian cells *(1)*. For the sake of simplicity, we refer to retroviral and lentiviral vectors as retroviridae-based vectors. This chapter describes a method for the transient production of high titer, helper-free retroviridae-based vectors *(4–6)*. The transient system for the production of retroviridae-based vectors is fast, reliable, and safe *(1,4,5)*. In fact, the transient nature of this system greatly minimizes the possible formation of replication-competent viruses, which may occur via homologous recombination *(1,4,5)*. The engineering of recombinant retroviridae vectors based on Moloney murine leukemia virus and HIV-1 is shown in **Figs. 1** and **2**, respectively *(7)*. Retroviridae vector stocks can be easily generated in 48 h after the transfection of packaging cells. Three plasmids are simultaneously co-transfected into the packaging cells: one plasmid encodes for the viral envelope, a second plasmid encodes for the components of the viral core (gag-pol), and a third plasmid contains the transgene of interest, which could be either a reporter gene, a therapeutic factor, or a combination of both. The function of the third plasmid consists in providing the chimerical viral genome for the packaging into the recombinant retroviridae-based vector. There are different systems to

From: *Methods in Molecular Biology, Vol. 285: Cell Cycle Control and Dysregulation Protocols*
Edited by: A. Giordano and G. Romano © Humana Press Inc., Totowa, NJ

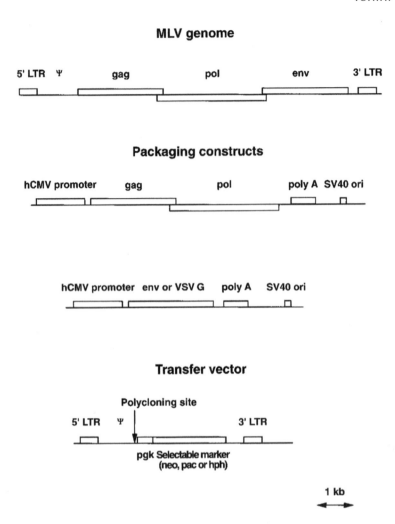

Fig. 1. Retroviral vector system based on the Moloney murine leukemia virus. Abbreviations: ψ = packaging signal; pgk = internal promoter driving the expression of a reporter gene or a selectable marker; neo = neomycin; pac = puromycin; hph = hygromycin; env = envelope; VSV-G = vesicular stomatitis virus G protein. Reproduced from **ref. 7** with permission, (www.stemcells.com).

co-transfect the three plasmids into the packaging cells. These systems are based on calcium phosphate precipitation, lipofectamine, chloroquine, and so on. We highly recommend relying on commercially available transfection reagents. The DNA transfection method described in this protocol is based on the classic calcium phosphate precipitation.

HIV-1 genome

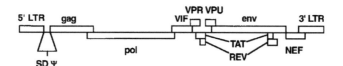

Packaging constructs

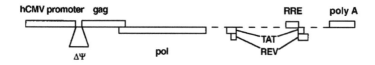

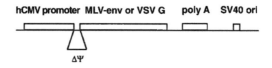

Transfer vector

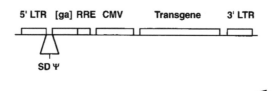

1 kb

Fig. 2. Lentiviral vector system based on HIV-1. Abbreviations: ψ = packaging signal; SD = splicing donor site; [ga] = initial sequence of gag gene; RRE = rev response element; MLV = murine leukemia virus; env = envelope; VSV G = vesicular stomatitis virus G protein. The accessory proteins (VIF, VPR, VPU, NEF) of HIV-1 have been deleted. The dashed line indicates the HIV-1 sequences that have been removed from the gag-pol packaging construct. Reproduced from **ref. 7** with permission.

The purpose of this chapter is only to provide investigators with the protocol to produce retroviridae-based vector stock. For safety guidelines, investigators must refer to and comply with the safety regulations provided by their institutions. The handling of retroviridae-based vectors requires particular safety procedures *(8)*. All institutions have guidelines available for investigators. A good reference for the handling of retroviridae-based vectors is *Biosafety in Microbiological and Biomedical Laboratories*, Third Edition (May 1993) HHS Pub. no. (CDC) 93-8395. U.S. Dept. of Health and Human Services, PHS, CDC, NIH. (*See also* http://www4.od.nih.gov/oba/guidelines.html for NIH guidelines to biomedical research.) In summary, the safety precautions require autoclaving of all solid waste (pipets, flasks, tissue culture dishes) and a 30-min treatment of liquid waste with chlorine bleach (e.g., Clorox) at a final 10% concentration in a closed plastic container. After this treatment, the liquid waste can be poured out into the sink. Lentiviral-based vectors may be handled in biosafety laboratories at containment 2 (BL2), but BL3 precautions must be taken.

2. Materials
2.1. Generation of Retroviridae-Producing Cell Line

1. Highly transfectable cell line, such as 293T cells.
2. Tissue culture material: dishes with a 10 cm diameter, flasks, pipets, tips.
3. Growth medium for packaging cells: Dulbecco's Modification of Eagle's Medium supplemented with 10% heat-inactivated fetal bovine serum, 100 U/mL penicillin, 100 U/mL streptomycin, 2 mM L-glutamine (*see* **Note 1**). Store at 4°C.
4. Freezing medium: 90% heat-inactivated fetal calf serum, 10% dimethyl sulfoxide.
5. 0.05% Trypsin-ethylenediamine tetraacetic acid (EDTA). Store at –20°C.
6. 2× *N*-hydroxyethylpiperazine-*N*′-2-ethanesulfonate-buffered saline (HBS): 50 mM *N*-hydroxyethylpiperazine-*N*′-2-ethanesulfonate, pH 7.1, 280 mM NaCl, 1.5 mM Na$_2$HPO$_4$. Store at –20°C for no longer than 6 mo (*see* **Note 2**).
7. 2 M CaCl$_2$. Store at –20°C for no longer than 6 mo (*see* **Note 2**).
8. Nuclease-free H$_2$O. Store at –20°C.
9. Vortex.

2.2. Retroviridae-Mediated Gene Tranfer into Target Cells

1. Target cells (*see* **Note 3**).
2. Retroviridae-based vector stocks.
3. Syringes.
4. Filters for syringes with 0.45-μm pore size membrane.
4. Polybrene at stock concentration of 4 mg/mL in PBS. Store at –20°C.

3. Method
3.1. Generation of Retroviridae-Producing Cell Line

1. Seed 2 × 10^6 293T-based cells in a 10-cm tissue culture dish in 10 mL of medium. Incubate at 37°C and 5% CO$_2$ for 24 h. The cells should reach 60% confluence at the time of transfection (*see* **Note 4**).
2. The next day, remove the medium from 293T cells and add 10 mL of fresh medium (*see* **Note 5**).

3. Thaw out the calcium phosphate reagents (2× HBS, $CaCl_2$, deionized H_2O) at room temperature (*see* **Note 6**).
4. Dispense 500 μL of 2× HBS in a 15-mL tissue culture tube.
5. In a second 15-mL tissue tube, dispense the three plasmids to generate the viral particles (*see* **Note 7**), 62 μL of $2M$ $CaCl_2$ and deionized H_2O to a final volume of 500 μL.
6. Add dropwise the DNA/calcium phosphate mixture to the 2× HBS solution while vortexing gently the 15-mL tissue culture tube. The mixture must not overflow.
7. Allow for the formation of the calcium phosphate precipitate by incubating the mixture for 30 min at room temperature, and by vortexing gently for 10 s every 10 min.
8. Take out the packaging cells from the incubator at the last moment. Add the mixture dropwise to the packaging cells. Gently rock the tissue culture dish and put back into the incubator.
9. Incubate the cells overnight at 37°C with 5% CO_2.
10. Check the packaging cells under the microscope the next morning. Small black particles should be visible under the microscope (*see* **Note 8**).
11. Change the medium and incubate the packaging cells in 10 mL of fresh medium at 37°C with 5% CO_2 for 24 h (*see* **Note 9**).
12. Harvest the supernatant from the packaging cells and filter it with 0.45-μm pore size filter (*see* **Note 10**). The supernatant containing the viral particles can be used for an immediate transduction or stored at –80°C for several months.

3.2. Retroviridae-Mediated Gene Transfer into Target Cells

1. Seed target cells (*see* **Notes 3** and **11**).
2. The day of transduction, remove the medium from the target cells and add 3 μL of polybrene at 4 mg/mL (*see* **Note 12**).
3. Infect the cells with 1 mL of viral supernatant and incubate overnight at 37°C (*see* **Note 12**).
4. Remove the supernatant containing the retroviridae-based vector and add fresh medium used for target cells.
5. The cells can be collected and analyzed after 24–48 h postinfection. As a first step, the cells should be analyzed for the expression of the reporter enzyme, such as *LacZ*, luciferase, green fluorescence protein, or antibiotic resistance (neomycin, puromycin, hygromycin, zeomycin; *see* **Note 11**).

4. Notes

1. Fetal bovine serum must be heat inactivated at 56°C for 30 min to destroy the complement. Retroviridae-based vectors are highly susceptible to complement-mediated lysis.
2. Avoid multiple freezing and thawing cycles. The thawing is carried out at room temperature. Vortex the tubes to achieve uniform mixing. Make single dose working aliquots after the first thawing. Store at –20°C.
3. Determine whether or not target cells can grow with the medium used for the packaging cells. Usually, established cell lines do not have any problem.

However, primary cells, embryonic stem cells, or somatic stem cells of various derivations may require certain growth factors. In this case, make 10× stocks of growth factors in order to supplement the medium of the retroviridae-based vectors at the time of the transduction. The calcium phosphate precipitation must be carried out in Dulbecco's Modified Eagle Medium-based medium, as the final pH of the reagents for the correct precipitation has been specifically determined for Dulbecco's Modified Eagle Medium. Retroviral vectors require cell division for gene transduction. Therefore, established cell lines should be split in a ratio of one to four the day before the retroviral transduction. Centrifugation is carried out at 200–240g for 5 min. Cells of hematopoietic lineage may require more time for centrifugation. Primary cells and stem cells of various derivations may require the addition of growth factors to stimulate cell division. However, stimulation of cell division may introduce cell culture artifacts *(1)*. In this respect, lentiviral-based vectors may be more useful, as they are able to transduce also nondividing cells. For this reason, there is no need to stimulate cell division. However, certain growth factors may still be needed for cell survival.

4. The density of 293T-based cells is a very critical parameter to achieve an efficient retroviridae-mediated gene transfer. Although 293T can be easily detached from the tissue culture dish, we recommend splitting 293T cells at room temperature with 0.05% trypsin-EDTA. 293T cells are usually grown in T-75 flasks with 20 mL of medium until they reach 70–80% confluence. The medium must be removed before adding 5 mL of 0.05% trypsin-EDTA. Incubate cells for 5 min at room temerature. Detach 293T cells by pipetting and dispense cell suspension in a 50-mL tissue culture tube containing 5 mL of complete medium. The presence of fetal bovine serum will neutralize trypsin. There is no need to centrifuge cells. However, if necessary, cells can be spun at 200–240g for 5 min. Cap the tissue culture tube and vortex gently for 5 s. Homogenize cell suspension by pipetting ten times and dispense 2 mL of cell suspension in tissue culture dishes containing 8 mL of medium. The optimal splitting ratio should be 1 to 5. It is important that 293T cells are seeded omogeneously and without too many clusters, in order to optimize DNA transfection efficiency. If 293T cells are seeded at low density, the viral titer will be too low. However, 293T cells must never reach confluence, otherwise they will begin to die. Of course, this will reduce the transduction efficiency. The degree of confluency of 293T cells must be 60% at the time of DNA co-transfection. The state of health of 293T cells must be optimal. The growth conditions of 293T cells are rather critical. 293T cells need to be split one to five or one to ten as they reach 70–80% confluence. If for any reason 293T should overgrow while they are in culture, discard them and thaw out a new vial of 293T cells. The number of passages of 293T cells seems to be also critical for efficient gene transduction. If the viral titer should decrease, discard the 293T cells and start a new culture. Usually, 293T cells should be kept in culture longer than 10 passages.

5. Cells generate metabolites while they are in culture. These metabolites, in turn, lower the pH of the medium, which will reduce the DNA transfection efficiency of the calcium phosphate. The change of the medium should be conducted 4 h prior to DNA transfection to allow for the equilibration of the pH of the medium in the CO_2 incubator at 37°C.

6. The reagents for the calcium phosphate kit must be gently thawed out at room temperature in the dark, as the 2× HBS solution is light sensitive. Make sure that the the reagents have reached room temperature before beginning the DNA transfection of 293T cells, as temperature affects the pH.

7. The dose of the three plasmids may vary according to the type of vector system. Dose-response assays should be conducted to optimize the viral titer. Usually, each plasmid concentration ranges from 10 to 20 μg. We recommend following the instructions reported in the literature per each gene delivery system.

8. The formation of the correct calcium phosphate precipitate is very critical. If the precipitate is too fine, the DNA transfection is not efficient. A fine precipitate is the result of a low pH at the time of the DNA transfection. In this case, check if the CO_2 incubator is working properly, recalibrate the pH meter if you have made your own calcium phosphate kit, make new reagents and check the quality of the growth medium. If the precipitate is too thick, most of the packaging cells will die. A thick precipitate is caused by a high pH. Also in this case you should check all the above-mentioned parameters. In addition, an old calcium phosphate kit may cause the formation of a thick precipitate, especially if the kit has been frozen and thawed several times.

9. It is very important to change the medium after the DNA transfection because the calcium phosphate precipitate is toxic to packaging cells. The medium must be changed very gently, as 293T cells have the tendency of detaching from the tissue culture dishes.

10. The time of harvesting may vary depending on the type of viral vector system being produced. Usually, lentiviral-based vectors require between 24 and 48 h incubation, whereas retroviral-based vectors may require between 48 and 72 h incubation. The optimal time of incubation should be determined by the investigator per each gene delivery system.

11. The amount of target cells depends on the scale of gene transduction and on the nature of the target cells. To determine the viral titer, target cells should be plated 24 h prior to transduction in 60-mm tissue culture dishes at a density ranging from 0.5 to 20×10^4. The assessment the titer of retroviridae-based vectors is described in other chapters. In order to engineer cell culture systems on a larger scale, we recommend using 10 mL of retroviridae-based vector supernatant per 2 to 5×10^6 target cells. The amount of polybrene required is 30 μL (3 μL per milliter of viral supernatant). However, we recommend not using polybrene, especially for primary and stem cell cultures.

12. The amounts of polybrene and viral supernant are referred to the titration of the retroviridae-based vector, which is carried out on a number of target cells ranging from 0.5 to 20×10^4, in a 60-mm tissue culture dish (*see* **Note 11**).

References

1. Romano, G., Micheli, P., Pacilio, C., and Giordano, A. (2000) Latest developments in gene transfer technology: achievements, perspectives, and controversies over therapeutic applications. *Stem Cells* **18,** 19–39.
2. Miller, D. G., Adam, M. A., and Miller, A. D. (1990) Gene transfer by retrovirus vector occurs only in cells that are replicating at the time of infection. *Mol. Cell Biol.* **10,** 4239–4242.
3. Poeschla, E., Corbeau, P. and Wong-Staal, F. (1996) Development of HIV vectors for anti-HIV gene therapy. *Proc. Natl. Acad. Sci. USA* **93,** 11,395–11,399.
4. Pear, W. S., Nolan, G.P., Scott, M. L., and Baltimore, D. (1993) Production of helper free retroviruses by transient transfection. *Proc. Natl. Acad. Sci. USA* **90,** 8392–8396.
5. Soneoka, Y., Cannon, P. M., Ramsdale, E. E., Griffiths, J. C., Romano, G., Kingsman, S. M., et al. (1995) A transient three-plasmid expression system for the production of high titer retroviral vectors. *Nucleic Acids Res.* **23,** 628–633.
6. Follenzi, A., Ailles, L. E., Bakovic, S., Geuna, M., and Naldini, L. (2000) Gene transfer by lentiviral vecotrs is limited by nuclear translocation and rescued by HIV-1 pol sequences. *Nat. Genet.* **25,** 217–222.
7. Romano, G., Pacilio, C., and Giordano, A. (1999) Gene transfer technology in therapy: current applications and future goals. *Stem Cells* **17,** 191–202.
8. Graham, F. L. and van der Eb, A. J. (1973) A new technique for the assay of infectivity of adenovirus 5 DNA. *Virology* **52,** 456–467.

19

Determination of Functional Viral Titer by Drug-Resistance Colony Assay, Expression of Green Fluorescent Protein, and β-Galactoside Staining

Tiziana Tonini, Pier Paolo Claudio, Antonio Giordano, and Gaetano Romano

1. Introduction

With this method, antibiotic selection of the infected cells gives rise to a countable number of colonies after 7-10 d *(1–4)*. Other reporter genes are based on green fluorescent protein (GFP; **ref.** *5*) or the *Escherichia coli lacZ* gene, which encodes for β-galactosidase for X-gal staining *(4,6)*. GFP-expressing cells can be easily visualized under an ultraviolet microscope. The main advantage is that GFP expression can be detected in living cells *(5)*. Retroviral and lentiviral transfer vectors can be engineered with an internal phosphoglycerate kinase (pgk) promoter driving the expression of a bacterial gene that confers resistance to a certain antibiotic *(1,2)*. Usually, the bacterial genes used are based on neomycin phosphotransferase, hygromycin B phosphotransferase, or puromycin *N*-acetyltransferase, which render mammalian cells resistant to G418, hygromycin B, and puromycin, respectively *(1)*. In addition, either the internal pgk or SV40 early promoter can drive the expression of *lacZ* gene *(4,6)* or GFP *(5)*. Functional titer does not provide a consistent measurement of virion concentration because it depends upon the transduction efficiency of the cell line being used to determine the titer. Therefore, several investigators use preferentially direct quantification for determining virus particle concentration. There are several bibliographic references for the counting of selected colonies *(3,4)*.

From: *Methods in Molecular Biology, Vol. 285: Cell Cycle Control and Dysregulation Protocols*
Edited by: A. Giordano and G. Romano © Humana Press Inc., Totowa, NJ

The purpose of this chapter is to provide investigators with the protocol to determine the titer of the retroviridae-based vector stock. For safety guidelines, investigators must refer and comply with the safety regulations provided by their institutions. For safety precautions, always wear two pairs of gloves, disposable lab coats, and use sterile barrier tips when working with retroviridae-based vectors. Treat all virus-containing liquid with chlorine bleach (e.g., Clorox) at a 10% final concentration for 20 min before discarding in the sink. Clean pipetman and working area with 10% chlorine bleach (e.g., Clorox) and with 70% ethanol at the end of the procedure. A good reference for retroviral vectors handling can be found in *Biosafety in Microbiological and Biomedical Laboratories*, Third Edition (May 1993) HHS Pub. no. (CDC) 93-8395. U.S. Dept. of Health and Human Services, PHS, CDC, NIH. (*See also* http://www4.od.nih.gov/oba/guidelines.html for NIH guidelines to biomedical research.) All institutions provide guidelines for the safe handling of potentially infectious agents. Investigators must comply with the safety guidelines.

2. Materials

2.1. Formation of Drug-Resistant Colonies

1. Mouse fibroblast NIH 3T3 cells.
2. Complete medium for NIH 3T3 cells: Dulbecco's Modified Eagle's Medium supplemented with 10% heat-inactivated fetal bovine serum and 2 mM L-glutamine (*see* **Note 1**). Store at 4°C.
3. Phosphate buffered saline (PBS): 37 mM NaCl, 2.7 mM KCl, 10 mM Na$_2$HPO$_4$, 1.4 mM KH$_2$PO$_4$, final pH 7.4. Store at 4°C.
4. Polybrene (Sigma H9268; *see* **Note 2**). Stock at 4 mg/mL in PBS. Store at –20°C.
5. Supernatant containing the retroviridae-based vector (*see* **Note 3**).
6. Antibiotic selection according to the resistance of the retroviridae-based transfer vector (*see* **Note 4**).
7. Trypsin 0.05%-ethylenediamine tetraacetic acid.
8. 0.3% Crystal Violet in 70% methanol.

2.2. Formation of GFP-Expressing Cells

1. *See* **Subheading 2.1., steps 1–7** (*see* **Note 3**).

2.3. Formation of β-Galactosidase-Positive Cells

1. *See* **Subheading 2.1., steps 1–5** (*see* **Note 3**).
2. 2% Formaldehyde and 0.2% gluteraldehyde in PBS. Prepare fresh each time.
3. X-gal (5-bromo-4-chloro-3-indolyl-β-D-galactopyranoside) dissolved in dimethyl sulfoxide at a concentration of 40 mg/mL. Store at –20°C.

4. 1 mg/mL X-gal (*see* **Subheading 2.3.**, **step 3**), 5 mM potassium ferricyanide, 5 mM potassium ferrocyanide, 2 mM MgCl$_2$ in PBS (*see* **Note 5**).

3. Methods

3.1. Formation of Drug-Resistant Colonies

1. Seed NIH 3T3 cells in a six-well plate 24 h before transfection at the density of 5 × 10^4 cells per well in complete medium (*see* **Note 6**). All centrifugation steps of NIH-3T3 cells are conducted at 200–240 g for 5 min.
2. Harvest retroviridae-based vector stock (*see* **Note 3**).
3. Prepare six 10-fold dilutions: set up six 1.5-mL sterile Eppendorf tubes and add 800 μL of complete medium to each tube. Add 200 μL of viral stock to the the first Eppendorf tube and mix by inverting several times. Transfer 200 μL from the first Eppendorf tube to the second one, discard the tip, and mix the contents of the tube by inverting several times. Repeat the procedure for all the remaining tubes, making sure to discard the tip after each transfer of viral supernatant.
4. Remove the medium from the six-well plates, add 3 μL of polybrene (at a stock of 4 mg/mL) in each well and the retroviridae-based vector contained in each Eppendorf tube. Remember to mark each well accordinglyas to not mismatch the various dilutions of viral supernatant. Gently rock the six-well plate and incubate overnight in a 5% CO$_2$ incubator at 37°C.
5. The next morning, remove the viral supernatant from the six-well plate, split cells 1:4 with trypsin (*see* **Note 7**) and incubate for 24 h in a 5% CO$_2$ incubator at 37°C.
6. At the end of the incubation, begin the antibiotic selection by replacing the medium with complete medium supplemented with the required antibiotic (*see* **Note 8**).
7. Usually, it takes around 7–10 d to obtain results.
8. Under the microscope, count the number of surviving colonies after all the mock control cells in the first well are dead and detached from the plate. Alternatively, cells can be fixed and stained with a 0.3% Crystal Violet solution in 70% methanol (*4*). The viral titer corresponds to the number of colonies present at the highest dilution that still contains colonies, multiplied by the diluition factor and by two, to account for the twofold increase in NIH 3T3 cells during the transduction period and the splitting 1:4. For example, three colony-forming units in the 10^6 dilution well correspond to a viral titer of 6 × 10^6 colony-forming U/mL.

3.2. Formation of GFP-Expressing Cells

1. *See* **Subheading 3.1.**, **steps 1–5** (*see* **Note 3**).
2. GFP expresion can be detected under the ultraviolet microscope on living cells. GFP-positive cells should appear between 24 and 48 h post-transduction. For the determination of the viral titer, *see* **Subheading 3.1.**, **step 8**.

3.3. Formation of β-Galactosidase-Positive Cells

1. *See* **Subheading 3.1.**, **steps 1–5** (*see* **Note 3**).
2. Wash three times NIH 3T3 cells with 5 mL of ice-cold PBS.

3. Fix cells for 5 min at room temperature with 5 mL of 2% formaldehyde and 0.2% gluteraldehyde in PBS.
4. Wash cells three times with 5 mL of ice-cold PBS.
5. Stain fixed cells at 4°C overnight with the following solution: 1 mg/mL X-gal, 5 mM potassium ferricyanide, 5 mM potassium ferrocyanide, and 2 mM MgCl$_2$ in PBS (*see* **Note 5**).
6. Count blue colonies under the microscope (**Subheading 3.1., step 8**).

4. Notes

1. Retroviral and lentiviral vector particles are susceptible to complement-mediated lysis. For this reason, the complement must be destroyed. Fetal bovine serum can be heat-inactivated at 56°C for 30 min. Heat-inactivated fetal bovine serum is also commercially available.
2. Polybrene is hexadimethrine bromide, a polycation that reduces charge repulsion between the virus and the cellular membrane.
3. The production of the supernatant containing the retroviridae-based vector has been described in another chapter (transient production of retroviral- and lentiviral-based vectors for the transduction of mammalian cells). By retroviridae we intend both retroviral and lentiviral-based vectors. Retroviridae-based vectors have been engineered to carry either an antibiotic resistance gene, *lacZ* gene, or GFP. The colony assay formation of antibiotic resistance is described in **Subheadings 2.1.** and **3.1.** The colony assay based on the detection of GFP-expressing cells is described in **Subheadings 2.2.** and **3.2.** The colony assay based on β-galactosidase staining is described in **Subheadings 2.3.** and **3.3.**
4. For NIH-3T3 cells the required amount of G418 is in the range of 1 mg/mL. The amount of puromycin is in the range of 600 μg/mL. The amount of hygromycin B is usually in the range of 1 mg/mL. The cell sensitivity to various antibiotics should be tested in dose response experiments, per each untransduced cell line, and per each batch of antibiotic. The incubation must be carried out in complete medium supplemented with various amounts of antibiotic, in a 5% CO$_2$ incubator, at 37°C. If cells die too rapidly (such as after an overnight incubation), the concentration of antibiotic is not suitable for the selection and should be lowered. Conversely, if cells tend to survive after 3 d, the concentration of antibiotic should be increased. Optimally, cells should begin to die after 24 h incubation with selective medium, and all cells should be dead after 72 h.
5. The β-galactoside hydrolyzing activity of the X-gal substrate generates a blue compound (*6*). This solution must be prepared fresh each time.
6. Retroviral vectors require cell division to access the chromosomal cellular DNA. For this reason, it is important to split NIH-3T3 cells 1:4 the day before retroviral transduction. Lentiviral vectors do not require cell division. However, it is better to seed NIH-3T3 cells at the right cell density, in order to avoid cell death caused by overgrowth.
7. To split cells 1:4, just add 2 mL of 0.05% trypsin-EDTA and incubate at 37°C for 5 min. At the end of the incubation, aspirate cell suspension, dispense in a 15-mL

sterile conical tube, add 2 mL of complete medium to inactivate trypsin, centrifuge at 200–240g for 5 min, remove the supernatant, resuspend with 8 mL of complete medium and dispense only 2 mL of cell suspension in a six-well plate.
8. Selective medium must be changed every 3 d.

References

1. Hawley, R. G., Lieu, F. H. L., Fong, A. Z. C., and Hawley, T. S. (1994) Versatile retroviral vectors for potential use in gene therapy. *Gene Ther.* **1,** 136–138.
2. Romano, G., Pacilio, C., and Giordano, A. (1999) Gene transfer technology in therapy: current applications and future goals. *Stem Cells* **17,** 191–202.
3. Pear, W. S., Nolan, G. P., Scott, M. L., and Baltimore, D. (1993) Production of helper free retroviruses by transient transfection. *Proc. Natl. Acad. Sci. USA* **90,** 8392–8396.
4. Soneoka, Y., Cannon, P. M., Ramsdale, E. E., Griffiths, J. C., Romano, G., Kingsman, S. M., et al. (1995) A transient three-plasmid expression system for the production of high titer retroviral vectors. *Nucleic Acids Res.* **23,** 628–633.
5. Cashion, L. M., Bare, L. A., Harvey, S., Trinh, Q., Zhu, Y., and Devlin, J. J. (1999) Use of enhanced green fluorescent protein to optimize and quantitate infection of target cells with recombinant retroviruses. *Biotechniques* **26,** 924-930.
6. Sane, J. R., Rubenstein, J. L. R., and Nicolas, J. F. (1986) Use of a recombinant retrovirus to study post-implantation cell lineage in mouse embryos. *EMBO J.* **5,** 3133–3142.

20

Retroviral and Lentiviral Vector Titration by the Analysis of the Activity of Viral Reverse Transcriptase

Tiziana Tonini, Pier Paolo Claudio, Antonio Giordano, and Gaetano Romano

1. Introduction

The assessment of the viral titer is an important step in optimizing and reproducing working conditions for the gene transduction for various mammalian cell types. The assessment of the viral titer is an important parameter to determine the maximum number of target cells that can be infected for a given volume of viral stock *(1)*.

This method provides a consistent measurement of virion concentration, as it depends upon the activity of viral reverse transcriptase contained by retroviral or lentiviral particles *(2)*. In this assay, the viral titer does not depend on the susceptibility of the target cell line to retroviral transduction. The reverse transcriptase assays reported in this protocol are suitable for retroviral vectors based on the Moloney murine leukemia virus and for lentiviral vectors based on the human immunodeficiency virus type 1 (HIV-1). The two vector systems have slightly different requirements for the buffers used to release the viral reverse transcriptase.

The purpose of this chapter is to provide investigators with the protocol to determine the titer of the retroviral- or lentiviral-based vector stocks. For safety guidelines, investigators must refer to and comply with the safety regulations provided by their institutions. For safety precautions, always wear two pairs of gloves, disposable lab coats, and use sterile barrier tips when working with retroviral- or lentiviral-based vectors. Treat all virus-containing liquid with chlorine bleach (e.g., Clorox) at a 10% final concentration for 20 min

From: *Methods in Molecular Biology, Vol. 285: Cell Cycle Control and Dysregulation Protocols*
Edited by: A. Giordano and G. Romano © Humana Press Inc., Totowa, NJ

before discarding in the sink. Clean pipetman and working area with 10% chlorine bleach (e.g., Clorox) and with 70% ethanol at the end of the procedure. A good reference for retroviral vector handling can be found in *Biosafety in Microbiological and Biomedical Laboratories*, Third Edition (May 1993) HHS Pub. no. (CDC) 93-8395. U.S. Dept. of Health and Human Services, PHS, CDC, NIH. (*See also* http://www4.od.nih.gov/oba/guidelines.html for NIH guidlines to biomedical research.) All institutions provide guidelines for the safe handling of potentially infectious agents. Investigators must comply with the safety guidelines. Also, for the handling and disposal of radioactive materials investigators must refer to guidelines provided by their institutions. These guidelines cannot be provided by our protocol.

2. Materials

2.1. Analyzing Moloney Murine Leukemia Virus Reverse Transcriptase by α[^{32}P]-Deoxythymidine Triphosphate (dTTP) Labeling

1. 1 M Tris-HCl, pH 8.
2. Nonidet P-40. Store at room temperature.
3. 1 M Dithiothreitol. Store at –20°C.
4. α[^{32}P]-dTTP at a specific activity of 1 Ci/mmol.
5. Oligodeoxythymidylic acid (oligo-dT, Pharmacia). Store at –20°C.
6. Polyriboadenylic acid·oligodT (poly(rA)·p(dT)$_{12-18}$; Pharmacia; *see* **Note 1**). Store at –20°C.
7. Reaction buffer: 50 mM Tris-HCl pH 8, 0.6 mM MnCl$_2$, 60 mM NaCl, 0.05% (v/v) Nonidet P-40, 20 mM dithiothreitol, 5 μg/mL oligo-dT, 10 μg/mL poly(rA)·p(dT)$_{12-18}$, 2 μCi of α[^{32}P]-dTTP (1 Ci/mmol). Prepare fresh each time.
8. Filters for syringes with 0.45-μm pore size.
9. Syringes.
10. Tissue culture material (96-well plates, flasks, pipets, and tissue culture dishes).
11. Packaging cell line producing retroviral vector particles (*see* **Note 2**).
12. Whatman DE81 filters.
13. 2× SSC solution: 0.3 M NaCl, 0.03 M sodium citrate, pH 7 (*see* **Note 3**).
14. 95% Ethanol.
15. Scintillation Cßounter Rackbeta 1214 (Wallac).

2.2. Analyzing HIV-1 Reverse Transcriptase by α[^{32}P]-dTTP Labeling

1. *See* **Subheading 2.1.**, steps 1–8.
2. dTTP.
3. Reaction buffer: 50 mM Tris-HCl pH 8, 10 mM MgCl$_2$, 0.75 mM MnCl$_2$, 60 mM NaCl, 0.05% (v/v) Nonidet P-40, 5 μg/mL oligo-dT, 10 μg/mL poly(rA)·p(dT)$_{12-18}$, 10 mM dTTP, 2 μCi of α[^{32}P]-dTTP (1 Ci/mmol; *see* **Note 4**). Prepare fresh each time.
4. *See* **Subheading 2.1.**, steps 10–17.

3. Methods

3.1. Analyzing Moloney Murine Leukemia Virus Reverse Transcriptase by α[^{32}P]-dTTP Labeling

1. Harvest 1 mL of supernatant containing retroviral vectors from a plate of packaging cells. Use a 1-mL syringe without needle.
2. Filter the retroviral supernatant through a 0.45-μm pore size membrane.
3. Mix in a 96-well plate 10 μL of filtered retroviral supernatant with 50 μL of reaction buffer and incubate at 37°C for 2 h.
4. Harvest 5 μL of reaction mixture and spot on a Whatman DE81 filter.
5. Let air dry for 10 min.
6. Wash the filter three times with gentle rocking at room temperature, for 10 min each time and with 500 mL of 2× SSC.
7. Wash the filter twice with 500 mL of 95% ethanol.
8. Let the filter dry at 37°C for 10 min.
9. The radioactivity can be measured with a scintillation counter Rackbeta 1214 (Wallac).

3.2. Analyzing HIV-1 Reverse Transcriptase by α[^{32}P]-dTTP Labeling

1. *See* **Subheading 3.2.**, **steps 1** and **2**.
2. Mix in a 96-well plate 25 μL of filtered lentiviral supernatant with 50 μL of reaction buffer and incubate at 37°C for 2 h.
3. Harvest 50 μL of reaction mixture (*see* **Subheading 3.2.**, **step 2**) and spot on a Whatman DE81 filter.
4. *See* **Subheading 3.1.**, **steps 5–9**.

4. Notes

1. Poly(rA)·p(dT)$_{12-18}$ is provided by Pharmacia in vials containing 5 U. Each unit of polymer corresponds roughly to 50 μg. The product comes as a lyophilized powder. Resuspend with nuclease-free water and store in small aliquots at –20°C.
2. The production of packaging cell lines for retroviral and lentiviral vectors has been described in another chapter. (Transient production of retroviral- and lentiviral-based vectors for the transduction of mammalian cells.)
3. SSC solution is stored at room temperature as 20× stock. The 2× SSC solution is freshly made each time by simply diluting the master stock 1:10 with nuclease-free water.
4. The reverse transcriptase of HIV-1 requires also $MgCl_2$.

References

1. Soneoka, Y., Cannon, P. M., Ramsdale, E. E., Griffiths, J. C., Romano, G., Kingsman, S. M., et al. (1995) A transient three-plasmid expression system for the production of high titer retroviral vectors. *Nucleic Acids Res.* **23,** 628–633.
2. Goff, S., Traktman, P., and Baltimore, D. (1981) Isolation and properties of Moloney leukemia virus mutants: use of a rapid assay for release of virion reverse transcriptase. *J. Virol.* **38,** 239–248.

V

DETECTION OF GENE EXPRESSION IN SUBCELLULAR COMPARTMENTS

21

Single and Double Colloidal Gold Labeling in Postembedding Immunoelectron Microscopy

Nicoletta Zini, Liliana Solimando, Caterina Cinti, and Nadir Mario Maraldi

1. Introduction

Immunocytochemistry is the most diffuse technique to visualize and localize specific biochemical components in cell compartments and tissues. With this method the antigens are tagged by antibodies that can be visualized with appropriate markers attached directly (direct method) or indirectly (indirect method) to them. The colloidal gold marker system *(1)* is the most widespread immuno-electron microscopy label for postembedding immunocytochemistry. Sections of embedded tissue are incubated with a primary antibody against a particular antigen, which is exposed on the surface of the section, and then with a secondary antibody conjugated to colloidal gold particles of a particular size (indirect method). It is possible to enlarge the colloidal gold size with silver enhancement. This technique is ideal for labeling both intracellular and surface antigens and it can be used for multiple labeling experiments and quantitative studies *(2)*.

A general problem in immunocytochemistry is to ensure both good ultra-structural preservation and well-retained antigenicity *(3)*. The method of fixation, the technique of tissue processing, and the choice of embedding agent are important factors in retaining tissue reactivity to antibodies. For these reasons it is suggested to use low concentration of glutaraldehyde (0.5–1.5%) or paraformaldehyde (2–4%) as fixative, avoid postfixation in osmium tetroxide, reduce the dehydration time, and polymerize at low temperature utilizing hydrophilic resins such as Lowicryl K4M *(3,4)* or London Resin White (LR White; **refs. 5** and **6**). LR White is compatible with about 12% by volume of

From: *Methods in Molecular Biology, Vol. 285: Cell Cycle Control and Dysregulation Protocols*
Edited by: A. Giordano and G. Romano © Humana Press Inc., Totowa, NJ

water, so that partial dehydration of tissue, which improves its reactivity particularly to antibodies, is made possible. However, it is possible to remove epoxy resins from the section with a solution of NaOH in ethanol or treat the Epon sections with H_2O_2 to make the sections more hydrophilic and the antigen unmasked. Moreover, in the case where the tissues are postfixed with osmium tetroxide, before immunolabeling, the sections can be incubated on a drop of saturated solution of sodium metaperiodate *(7)*.

The success of the immunolabeling depends on the quality of the primary antibody used. The monoclonal or polyclonal antibody should be of good specificity and high affinity. It should be directed against a highly purified and well-characterized antigen and the interaction should be assessed through immunochemical techniques. The optimal dilution of the primary antibody corresponds to that giving the highest labeling and the lowest background. To avoid nonspecific adsorption on sections of immunoreagents it is suggested to use buffers containing bovine serum albumin (BSA) in all the incubation steps and to treat the sections with nonimmune serum from the species which produced the secondary antibody (i.e., normal goat serum if the secondary antibody has been obtained in goat). Controls consist of samples not incubated with the primary antibody or incubated with nonimmune serum.

The aim of this chapter is to describe the processing methods currently used for single (**Fig. 1**) or double (**Figs. 2** and **3**) colloidal gold labeling in postembedding immunoelectron microscopy. The samples are fixed, dehydrated, and embedded in Epon or in LR White resin. Thin sections obtained by ultramicrotomy, are picked up on nickel grids, immunolabeled, stained, and observed by electron microscopy.

2. Materials

2.1. Preparation of Cell and Tissue Sections

1. Phosphate-buffered saline (PBS): 37 mM NaCl, 2.7 mM KCl, 10 mM Na$_2$HPO$_4$, 1.4 mM KH$_2$PO$_4$, pH 7.4 (*see* **Note 1**).
2. 0.25% (v/v) Trypsin, 1 mM ethylenediamine tetraacetic acid in PBS.
3. 0.2 M Phosphate buffer, pH 7.2 (Sörensen): 100 mL of 0.2 M phosphate buffer, pH 7.2 (method of Sörensen) are obtained by mixing 72 mL of 0.2 M dibasic sodium phosphate solution and 28 mL of 0.2 M monobasic sodium phosphate solution.
4. Polypropylene tubes (*see* **Note 2**).
5. Fixing solution: 1% (v/v) glutaraldehyde, electron microscopy (EM) grade in 0.1 M phosphate buffer, pH 7.2: prepare 50 mL of 1% (v/v) glutaraldehyde by mixing 25 mL of 0.2 M phosphate buffer, pH 7.2; 2 mL of 25% (v/v) glutaraldehyde in H$_2$O (EM grade; Fluka, Buchs, Switzerland); and 23 mL of bidistilled water (H$_2$O). Store at 4°C in the dark. The solution should appear clear. Do not use if it appears yellow.

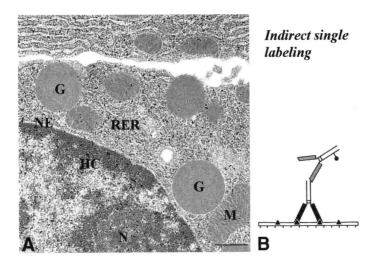

Indirect single labeling

Fig. 1. Indirect single labeling in postembedding electron microscopy. (**A**) Section of rat pancreas fixed with 1% (v/v) glutaraldehyde and embedded in Epon 812. The section is incubated with the primary antibody, the mouse KT10 monoclonal anti-phosphatidylinositol 4,5 bisphosphate, diluted 1:100 (v/v), and then with the secondary antibody, a goat anti-mouse conjugated to 10-nm colloidal gold particles (GAM IgG 10 nm). Gold particles are amplified 4 min with a Silver Enhancer Kit (Amersham Life Science). In the cytoplasm, the labeling is found along the rough endoplasmic reticulum (RER); the zymogen granules (G) and mitochondria (M) are unlabeled. In the nucleus, besides the nuclear envelope (NE), the heterochromatin (HC) is highly labeled. N, nucleolus. Bar = 0.5 μm. (**B**) Scheme of the single labeling procedure.

6. Fixing solution: 4% (w/v) paraformaldehyde in 0.1 M phosphate buffer, pH 7.2: prepare 25 mL of 8% (w/v) paraformaldehyde solution by dissolving 2 g of paraformaldehyde powder in 20 mL of H_2O and heating to 65°C with stirring. Add a few drops of 1 N NaOH, with continued stirring, until the solution becomes clear. Make up to 25 mL with H_2O and allow the solution to cool. Filter through a 0.22-μm filter. Prepare the fixative with 25 mL of 8% (w/v) paraformaldehyde in H_2O and 25 mL of 0.2 M phosphate buffer, pH 7.2. Store at 4°C for a few days.
7. Washing solution: 0.15 M phosphate buffer, pH 7.2.
8. Graded series up to absolute ethanol: 50, 70, 90, and 100% (v/v).
9. Propylene oxide (*see* **Note 3**).
10. Epon embedding medium: epon embedding medium is obtained by mixing 20 mL of A mixture (62 mL Epon 812 and 100 mL dodecenyl succinic anhydride) and 10 mL of B mixture (100 mL Epon 812 and 89 mL methyl nadic anydride). Add 0.45 mL of Tris-(dimethylaminomethyl)-phenol. Epoxy resin components

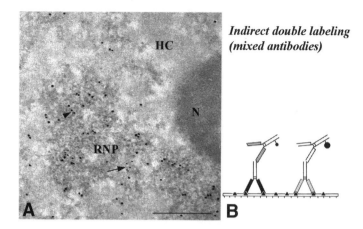

Fig. 2. Mixed antibodies indirect double labeling in postembedding electron microscopy. **(A)** Section of Saos-2 cells fixed with 1% (v/v) glutaraldehyde, partially dehydrated and embedded in LR White at 0°C. The section is incubated with a mixture of primary antibodies, the anti-SC35 splicing factor mouse monoclonal antibody and the anti-PLCβ$_1$ rabbit polyclonal antibody, final dilution 1:5 and 1:50, respectively. The antibodies are revealed by a mixture of the secondary antibodies: a goat anti-mouse conjugated to colloidal gold particles of 10 nm (arrow) and a goat anti-rabbit conjugated to colloidal gold particles of 30 nm (arrowhead). The double labeling are present on the ribonucleoprotein particle clusters (RNP) in the nucleus of Saos-2 cells. HC, heterochromatin. Bar = 0.5 μm. **(B)** Scheme of mixed antibodies double labeling procedure.

can be purchased from companies, which are specialized in EM reagent supply (i.e., from Polysciences, Warrington, PA).

11. LR White embedding medium and accelerator for LR White (*see* **Note 4**).
12. Diamond knife for ultramicrotomy.
13. Nickel EM grids (*see* **Note 5**).

2.2. Immunolabeling

1. 10% (v/v) H_2O_2 for Epon sections only.
2. 0.5 *M* Tris buffer, pH 7.6: dissolve 60.57 g of Tris powder [Tris (hydroxymethyl)-aminomethane] in H_2O, adjust the pH to 7.6 with 1 *N* HCl, and make up to 1000 mL with H_2O. It can be stored in small aliquots at –20°C.
3. 0.2 *M* Tris buffer, pH 8.2: dissolve 24.228 g of Tris powder in H_2O, adjusting the pH to 8.2 with 1 *N* HCl, and make up to 1000 mL with H_2O. It can be stored in small aliquots at –20°C.
4. TBS I solution: 0.05 *M* Tris buffer saline, pH 7.6, supplemented with 0.1% (w/v) bovine serum albumin (BSA): 0.5 *M* Tris 1:10 (v/v) with 0.9% (v/v) NaCl plus 0.1% (w/v) BSA for blocking nonspecific binding. Freshly prepared TBS I is rec-

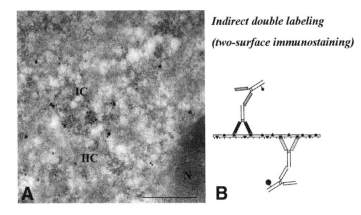

Indirect double labeling

(two-surface immunostaining)

Fig. 3. Two-surface indirect double labeling in postembedding electron microscopy. **(A)** Section of Saos-2 cells fixed with 1% (v/v) glutaraldehyde, partially dehydrated and embedded in LR White at 0°C. Double labeling by two-surface immunostaining is used when the two primary antibodies are of the same species. In the first step the grid is incubated on one side with anti-pRb2/p130 retinoblastoma protein rabbit polyclonal antibody, diluted 1:50 (v/v), and a goat anti-rabbit 5 nm colloidal gold; in the second step, the incubation is performed on the other face of the grid with anti-E2F4 transcription factor rabbit polyclonal antibody diluted 1:20 (v/v), and a goat anti-rabbit 15 nm colloidal gold. Gold particles were amplified 4 min with Silver Enhancer Kit. The double labelings are particularly evident in interchromatin domains (IC). HC, heterochromatin. Bar = 0.5 μm. **(B)** Scheme of two-surface immunolabeling procedure.

ommended. If 0.1% (w/v) BSA is not sufficient to reduce or eliminate nonspecific labeling, it is possible to incubate the grid with a solution constituted by 3% (w/v) nonfat dry milk and 2% (w/v) BSA in TBS I for 1 h and 30 min at room temperature before nonimmune serum.

5. TBS II solution: 0.02 M Tris buffer saline, pH 8.2, supplemented with 0.1% (w/v) BSA; Dilute 0.2 M Tris 1:10 (v/v) with 0.9% (v/v) NaCl plus 0.1% (w/v) BSA. Freshly prepared TBS II is recommended.
6. Nonimmune serum 1:20 (v/v) in TBS I (*see* **Note 6**).
7. Primary antibody diluted in TBS I (*see* **Note 7**).
8. Gold-conjugated secondary antibody, directed against the primary antibody, diluted 1:10 (v/v) in TBS II. Store at 4°C (*see* **Note 8**).
9. Silver enhancement kit (*see* **Note 9**).
10. 3% (v/v) Uranyl acetate in 50% (v/v) ethanol and 3% (v/v) uranyl acetate in bidistilled water (H₂O; *see* **Note 10**).
11. Lead citrate (Reinolds, *see* **Note 11**)
12. Carbon coating for LR White sections (*see* **Note 12**).

3. Methods

3.1. Preparation of Cell and Tissue Sections

1. Wash with ice-cold PBS the pellets obtained by centrifugation (400g, 5 min) of about 10×10^6 cells.
2. Cells or tissues (1 mm^3 size) are fixed with 1% (v/v) glutaraldehyde or 4% (w/v) paraformaldehyde for 1 h at 4°C.
3. Quickly rinse the samples three times with 0.15 M phosphate buffer and once again overnight at 4°C.
4. Divide the cell pellet or tissue in distinct tubes and include in Epon and/or in LR White.
5. Dehydration and Epon embedding: dehydrate the samples in 70% (v/v) ethanol for three times, 10 min each; in 90% (v/v) ethanol for three times, 10 min each; and in 100% (v/v) ethanol for three times, 10 min each. Treat twice for 15 min each with propylene oxide. Infiltrate the samples in 1:1 (v/v) mixture Epon/propylene oxide for 1 h, then in 3:1 (v/v) overnight. Infiltrate in Epon for 2 h. All the steps are performed at room temperature. Polymerize 48 h at 60°C.
6. Dehydration and LR White embedding: dehydrate in 50% (v/v) ethanol 15 min, in 70% (v/v) ethanol twice for 15 min, infiltrate with 2:1 (v/v) mixture LR White/70% (v/v) ethanol 30 min, then in pure LR White four times for 20 min each. If possible, use gentle agitation on a rotary device at room temperature. Polymerize LR White mixed with accelerator at 0°C in ice bath. Quickly fill the tube and cap, and place in refrigerator at 0°C for 3 h or overnight.
7. Cut the embedded samples with a diamond knife at the ultramicrotome: 90-nm Epon thin sections and 110-nm LR White thin sections.
8. Pick up the sections on nickel EM grids.

3.2. Immunolabeling

3.2.1. Single Labeling (**Fig. 1**)

1. Prepare a series of droplets of each reagent used on a Parafilm strip. The grids may be floated or fully immersed in the droplets. Never leave the grids to dry during incubation.
2. Only for Epon sections: treat the grids with 10% (v/v) H_2O_2 by floating sections on the droplet for 3 min, then deep them completely for 7 min. Rinse six times in H_2O.
3. Epon and LR White sections are washed twice in TBS I for 5 min each.
4. Incubate with 1:20 nonimmune serum in TBS I for 30 min in a wet box.
5. Incubate with the primary antibody diluted in TBS I overnight at 4°C.
6. Wash six times with TBS I for 2 min each.
7. Wash twice with TBS II for 2 min each.
8. Incubate with the secondary antibody conjugated with colloidal gold particles diluted 1:10 (v/v) in TBS II for 1 h in a wet box, in the dark and at room temperature.
9. Wash six times with TBS II for 2 min each.
10. Wash three times with H_2O for 2 min each.
11. Intensify with silver enhancement kit, if necessary.

12. Rinse well with H_2O.
13. Dry with filter paper.
14. For Epon sections, stain 15 min with alcoholic uranyl acetate; for LR White sections, stain 5 min with aqueous uranyl acetate (*see* **Subheading 2.2., step 10**). Rinse well with H_2O and stain with lead citrate 15 min for Epon and 2 min for LR White. Rinse well with H_2O.
15. Carbon coating for LR White sections.

3.2.2. Double Labeling

3.2.2.1. MIXED SPECIES IMMUNOGOLD (PRIMARY ANTIBODIES OF DIFFERENT SPECIES; **FIG. 2**)

1–4. *See* **Subheading 3.2.1., steps 1–4**.
  5. Incubation with a mixture of primary antibodies diluted in TBS I overnight at 4°C.
6–7. *See* **Subheading 3.2.1., steps 6** and **7**.
  8. Incubation with a mixture of the secondary antibodies conjugated with colloidal gold particles of different size, final dilution 1:10 (v/v) in TBS II for 1 h at room temperature in the dark.
9–15. *See* **Subheading 3.2.1., steps 9–15**.

3.2.2.2. TWO-SURFACE IMMUNOSTAINING (PRIMARY ANTIBODIES OF THE SAME SPECIES; **FIG. 3**)

  1. In this procedure the grids must be floated at all stages.
2–10. *See* **Subheading 3.2.1., steps 2–10**
 11. Dry with filter paper.
 12. The grid must be floated section upside-down (*see* **Note 13**).
 13. Repeat the same procedure as **steps 2–10** in **Subheading 3.2.1.** for second antigen detection.
 14. *See* **Subheading 3.2.1., steps 11–15**.

4. Notes

 1. Stable at room temperature.
 2. Polypropylene tubes (1.3 cm diameter and 5.6 cm height) are recommended for fixation and embedding procedure.
 3. Propylene oxide is used routinely in between ethanol dehydration and infiltration with epoxy resin embedding media.
 4. LR White is used pure during infiltration and with accelerator (1.5 µL/mL) during the embedding at 0°C. LR White is a hydrophilic resin suitable for immunoelectron microscopy because it allows a partial dehydration and low polymerization temperatures. LR White and its accelerator can be purchased from companies that specialize in EM reagent supply (i.e., from Polysciences).
 5. Nickel or gold grids are recommended because do not react with immunogold reagents. The grids can be purchased from companies, which are specialized in EM reagent supply (i.e., from Balzers, Fürstentum, Liechtenstein).

6. Nonimmune serum from the species that produced the secondary antibody is rec-ommended to avoid nonspecific adsorption of immunoreagents on sections (i.e., normal goat serum if the secondary antibody has been obtained in goat).

7. Determine the monoclonal or polyclonal source of the antibody, the animal species used, and the subclass it belongs to for the choice of the secondary antibody. Test the best dilution.

8. Secondary antibodies are available conjugated to colloidal gold with different par-ticle sizes (5, 10, 20, and 30 nm) by specialized companies (i.e., Amersham Life Science, Bio Cell Research Laboratories, Cardiff, UK). The most used colloidal gold size in postembedding immunoelectron microscopy is 10 nm.

9. It is possible to enlarge the colloidal gold size by using Silver Enhancement Kit, ready to use. Prepare the Silver Enhancement reagent by mixing equal drops of reagents A and B in a small tube immediately prior to use. Silver Enhancement Kit can be purchased from specialized companies (i.e., Amersham Life Science).

10. 3% (v/v) Uranyl acetate is prepared by 6% (w/v) uranyl acetate stock solution in H_2O obtained by dissolving 6 g of powder in 100 mL of H_2O. Store at 4°C. It is used for grid staining. Uranyl acetate powder can be purchased from companies that specialize in EM reagent supply (i.e., from Electron Microscopy Sciences, Fort Washington, PA).

11. Lead citrate is obtained by mixing 1.33 g of lead nitrate with 1.76 g of sodium cit-rate and 30 mL of H_2O. Stir for 30 min, add 8.0 mL of 1 N NaOH, and dilute the suspension to 50 mL with H_2O. Filter trough a 0.22-μm filter. Store at 4°C. The solution is used for grid staining.

12. This step is suggested, but not essential. The carbon coating stabilizes the samples embedded in the hydrophilic resin LR White. It is performed in an evaporation unit such as Edwards Coating System E306A (Edwards High Vacuum International, Wilmington, MA).

13. Alternatively, it is possible to incubate the grids for the second antigen detection on the same surface after fixation with 1% (v/v) or 2% (v/v) glutaraldehyde in 0.1 M phosphate buffer for 30 min at 4°C. After this treatment no cross-reactivity occurs between the first and the second immunoreagent.

References

1. Hayat, M. A. ed. (1989) *Colloidal Gold: Principles, Methods, and Applications*, Vols. 1–3, Academic Press, San Diego, California.

2. Zini, N., Trimarchi, C., Claudio, P. P., Stiegler, P., Marinelli, F., Maltarello, M. C., et al. (2001) pRb2/p130 and p107 control cell growth by multiple strategies and in asso-ciation with different compartments within the nucleus. *J. Cell. Physiol.* **189,** 34–44.

3. Bendayan, M., Nanci, A., and Kan, F. W. K. (1987) Effect of tissue processing on colloidal gold cytochemistry. *J. Histochem. Cytochem.* **35,** 983–996.

4. Altman, L. G., Schneider, B. G., and Papermaster, D. S. (1984) Rapid embedding of tissues in Lowicryl K4M for immunoelectron microscopy. *J. Histochem. Cytochem.* **32,** 1217–1223.

5. Newman, G. R. and Hobot, J. A. (1987) Modern acrylics for post-embedding immunostaining techniques. *J. Histochem. Cytochem.* **35,** 971–981.
6. Zini, N., Sabatelli, P., Faenza, I., Ognibene, A., and Maraldi, N. M. (1996) Interleukin 1α induces variation of the intranuclear amount of phosphatidylinositol 4,5-bisphosphate and phospholipase Cβ₁ in human osteosarcoma Saos-2 cells. *Histochem. J.* **28,** 495–504.
7. Bendayan, M. and Zollinger, M. (1983) Ultrastructural localization of antigenic sites on osmium-fixed tissues applying the protein A-gold technique. *J. Histochem. Cytochem.* **31,** 101–109.

22

Multifluorescence Labeling and Colocalization Analyses

Massimo Riccio, Maja Dembic, Caterina Cinti, and Spartaco Santi

1. Introduction

The fluorescence labeling technique is a method with a high degree of specificity and sensitivity and is often chosen as a tool in the study of protein expression and subcellular compartments (*1*). Recently, a large number of fluorescent dyes with distinct fluorescence excitation and emission spectra have been engineered to be used in multilabeling and co-localization experiments. Some of the most common fluorescent dyes are fluorescein isothiocyanate (FITC), Cy2, Cy3, Cy5, TRITC, and rhodamine. These dyes can be excited independently using different laser wavelengths and observed in separate fluorescent channels. The efficiency of the fluorescent probes is, however, hampered by a variable degree of spectral overlap, low quantum efficiencies and extinction coefficients, or rapid photobleaching.

Two different antibodies, conjugated with two different fluorochromes (i.e., FITC-conjugated antibody: green fluorescence; Cy5-conjugated antibody: far red fluorescence) are used in double-fluorescence labeling. Because of their distinct excitation and emission spectra, they can be easily distinguished from each other when observed at an optical epifluorescence microscope.

Analyses with double-fluorescent labeling, such as three-dimensional reconstructions and/or quantification, require a sensitive detection system capable of resolving multiple fluorescent signals in a very accurate way. A general method for the imaging technique takes advantage of the particular properties of confocal laser scanning microscope (CLSM), which performs an optical sectioning of the sample by rejection of the out-of-focus light via a confocal pinhole. This feature makes possible the scanning of different x–y

From: *Methods in Molecular Biology, Vol. 285: Cell Cycle Control and Dysregulation Protocols*
Edited by: A. Giordano and G. Romano © Humana Press Inc., Totowa, NJ

planes along the *z*-axis, corresponding to different depths of the sample. Afterwards, by ordering the planes into a vertical stack, a three-dimensional image of the specimen can be reconstructed. Because it does not require physical sectioning of thick samples and precludes the need for extensive specimen processing, CLSM is one of the most efficient methods available to measure multiple fluorescent signals and gain three-dimensional information from the specimens (**Fig. 1**; **refs. *2*** and ***3***).

Double-immunofluorescence detection must be accurate to perform precise colocalization analysis. This can only occur if emission spectra of the fluorochromes are sufficiently separated and the correct filter sets are being used during the acquisition step by CLSM. To this aim, red and green wavelengths are usually selected to excite the fluorochromes at their maximum excitation peak, while a good degree of separation between the emission wavelengths is still maintained (*see* **Subheading 3.2.**).

The colocalization degree of the fluorochromes can be measured by comparing the equivalent pixel positions between the acquired images. Afterwards, a scatterplot of the individual pixels from the paired images is generated (**Fig. 2A–C**). Dimmer pixels in the image are located toward the origin of the scatterplot, while brighter pixels are located farther out. Pure red and pure green pixels tend to cluster more toward the corresponding axes of the plot. If colocalized pixels are present, they appear as orange to yellow, depending on the degree of colocalization, toward the middle of the plot (*4,5*).

A more quantitative assessment of the colocalized areas can be performed using colocalization coefficients calculated for pixel values contained within the region of interest (ROI): Pearson's correlations (R_p), k_1, and k_2 coefficients, overlap coefficient (R; *6* and *7*). Pearson's correlation provides information about the similarity of shape between images and does not take into account image intensity (spatial colocalization). It is a value computed to be between -1 and 1. Coefficients k_1 and k_2 describe the differences in intensities of red and green ($R^2 = k_2 \cdot k_2$). The value k_1 is sensitive to differences in intensity for green, whereas k_2 is sensitive to differences in intensity for red. The overlap coefficient is simultaneously used to describe colocalization: this method does not perform any pixel averaging functions, so correlations are returned as values between 0 and 1. This method is not sensitive to intensity variations in the image analysis. This is especially important when considering issues typical to fluorescence imaging such as sample photo-bleaching or different setting of the detectors. An example of co-localization coefficient values for the coimmunostaining is shown in **Table 1**.

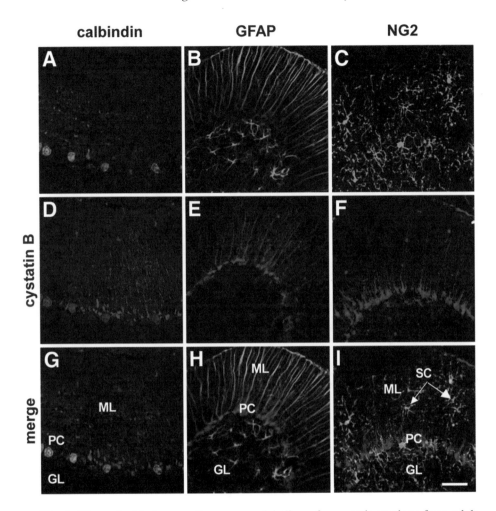

Fig. 1. Three double-immunofluorescence labeling of cryostatic sections from adult rat cerebellum. The anti-Calbindin FITC-conjugated antibody (green immunofluorescence) is intense in the Purkinje's cells (**A**); on the contrary, anti-cystatin B Cy5-conjugated antibody (red immunofluorescence) is detectable not only in the Purkinje's cells but also in small cells of the molecular layer (**D**). The merging of the two signals shows the overlapping of green and red fluorescence, generating a yellow color (**G**). In (**B**) the green immunofluorescence of anti-GFAP antibody is strongly detectable in the astrocytes of the cerebellar glia. In (**E**) the immunostaining of the same field with antibody against cystatin B is shown; in (**H**) the merging image of (**B**) and (**E**) is shown. **C** shows the immunocytochemical localization of NG2: basket, Golgi, stellate, and oligodendrocyte progenitor cells. The red immunofluorescence indicates cystatin B in (**F**) and the merging of (**C**) and (**F**) in (**I**). ML, molecular layer; GL, granule layer; PC, Purkinje's cells; SC, stellate cells. Bar = 40 µm.

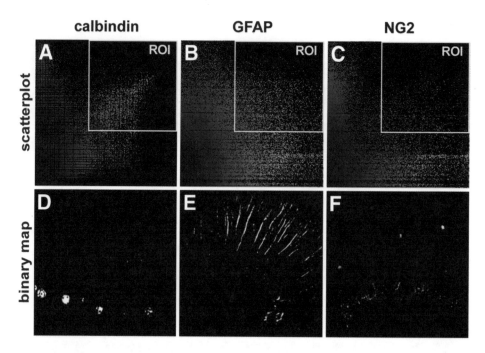

Fig. 2. Colocalization analysis of three double-immunofluorescence labeling. Colocalization of the fluorescence signals is colored in yellow and localized on the diagonal area of the scatterplots (**A–C**). An ROI is drawn in yellow on the scatterplots to indicate the following areas of analysis. The binary maps presented in (**D**), (**E**), and (**F**) show regions in which the two signals are present together above a defined threshold of fluorescence intensity.

Table 1
Quantification of the Colocalized Fluorescent Signals

	calbindin–cystatin B	GFAP–cystatin B	NG2–cystatin B
Pearson's correlations (R_p)	0.38	0.28	0.13
Coefficient k_1	1.50	0.53	0.14
Coefficient k_2	0.45	0.43	0.46
Overlap coefficient (R)	0.69	0.48	0.25

The values indicated for the correlation coefficients are calculated from the images shown in **Fig. 1.**

2. Materials

1. Phosphate-buffered saline (PBS): 37 mM NaCl, 2.7 mM KCl, 10 mM Na$_2$HPO$_4$, 1.4 mM KH$_2$PO$_4$, pH 7.4.
2. Fixing solutions: 4% (w/v) paraformaldehyde in PBS.
3. Fixing/cryoprotection solutions: 4% (w/v) paraformaldehyde, 10% (w/v) sucrose in PBS.
4. Cryoprotection solutions: 10% (w/v) sucrose in PBS.
5. Iso-pentane (Riedel-de Haen).
6. Permeabilization solution: 0.1% (w/v) Triton X100 in PBS.
7. Blocking solutions: 3% (w/v) bovine serum albumin in PBS.
8. Primary antibodies: monoclonal or polyclonal.
9. Secondary antibodies: conjugated with fluorochromes (FITC, Cy2, Cy3, Cy5, TRITC, rhodamine).
10. Antifading solution: 0.21 M 1,4-diazabicyclo-[2.2.2]octane (Sigma, St Louis, MO), 90% (w/v) glycerol in 0.02 M Tris-HCl, pH 8.0.
11. Optical Epifluorescence Microscope (Nikon TE300), equipped with a plan-apochromat Nikon 60×, 1.40 N.A. oil-immersion objective.
12. Confocal Microscope Radiance 2000 (Bio-Rad, Hercules, CA) equipped with a plan-apochromat Nikon 60×, 1.40 N.A. oil-immersion objective, an argon/krypton, and a red diode laser.
13. LaserPix Software (Bio-Rad).
14. ImageSpace Software (Molecular Dynamics, Mountain View, CA) running on a workstation Indigo2 (Silicon Graphics, Mountain View, CA).

3. Methods

3.1. Multifluorescence Labeling

1. The samples are usually dissected, post-fixed in 150 mL of fixing/cryoprotection solution for 2 h at 4°C, maintained in cryoprotection solution for at least 1 h at 4°C and frozen in iso-penthane (*see* **Subheading 3**, **step 5**) cooled in liquid nitrogen.
2. Cut the frozen sample by cryostat in 10-μm sections (*see* **Note 1**).
3. Wash in PBS.
4. Incubate the sections with permeabilization solution for 5 min at room temperature.
5. Incubate with blocking solution for 30 min at room temperature.
6. Incubate with a mixture of primary antibodies (*see* **Note 2**) diluted 1:50 in blocking solution (*see* **Subheading 3**, **step 7**) for 1 h at room temperature.
7. Wash in blocking solution.
8. Incubate with a mixture of secondary antibodies (*see* **Notes 2** and **3**) diluted 1:50 (v/v) in blocking solution for 1 h at room temperature.
9. Wash with PBS.
10. Add on the sections 10 μL of anti-fading solution.
11. Mount the specimens with a cover slide.
12. Observe the samples at optical epifluorescent microscope, or at CLSM to gain the images, three-dimensional information and quantify the co-localization of the fluorescent signals.

3.2. CLSM Imaging

1. Use laser wavelength that corresponds to the maximum excitation peak of the flu-orochrome in use (i.e., 488 nm wavelength of an argon/krypton laser to excite FITC and 637 nm of a red diode laser to excite Cy5).
2. Set the power of the laser at a medium level to avoid photobleaching (i.e., argon/krypton laser at 20% and red diode laser at 30%).
3. Detect in sequential mode to separate completely the emission wavelengths of the two fluorochromes.
4. Use filters for the emission bands to get the maximum separation of the signals (i.e., a band pass filter BP: 515/530 to acquire the green emission of FITC and a long pass filter LP660 to detect the far red emission of Cy5).
5. Acquire serial sections along the *z*-axis of the sample with an increment step of 0.5 μm.
6. Perform the volume rendering by ImageSpace Software.

3.3. Colocalization Analyses by CLSM

1. Construct a scatterplot of the image using the ImageSpace Software (*see* **Subheading 2, step 14**) .
2. Select a ROI on the scatterplot that contains an area with intensity values upper to threshold levels (*see* **Note 4**).
3. Calculate the colocalization map (binary image) using ImageSpace Software for the selected ROI.
4. Calculate the values of the following coefficients with LaserPix Software to obtain a more quantitative evaluation of the co-localization:

$$\text{Pearson's correlations } (R_p) = \frac{\sum_i (S1_i - S1_{aver}) \cdot (S2_i - S2_{aver})}{\sqrt{\sum_i (S1_i - S1_{aver})^2 \cdot \sum_i (S2_i - S2_{aver})^2}}$$

$$\text{coefficient } k_1 = \frac{\sum_i S1_i \cdot S2_i}{\sum_i (S1_i)^2}$$

$$\text{coefficient } k_2 = \frac{\sum_i S1_i \cdot S2_i}{\sum_i (S1_i)^2}$$

$$\text{Overlap coefficient } (R)^2 = k_1 \cdot k_2$$

i = voxel
$S1$ = grey value of the first signal
$S2$ = grey value of the second signal
$S1_{aver}$ = average value of $S1_i$
$S2_{aver}$ = average value of $S2_i$

4. Notes

1. Mount the sections on Silane-prep™ slides (Sigma).
2. Double labeling cannot be performed if crossreactions between the antibodies are present. Therefore, try to choose the combination of monoclonal and polyclonal antibodies, or when this is impossible (i.e., both monoclonal or both polyclonal) try to choose two antibodies produced by different hosts.
3. The fluorochromes, conjugated to the secondary antibodies, must be selected to avoid overlaps between the excitation and emission wavelengths; that is, Cy5-conjugated (ex: 650 nm, em: 670 nm) and FITC-conjugated (ex: 488 nm, em: 520 nm).
4. Try to avoid signals lower then 150 levels of gray to exclude background and select only highly colocalized fluorochromes.

Acknowledgments

We are grateful to Dr. Patrizia Ambrogini for help in animal care and Dr. William Stallcup for the generous gift of anti-NG2 antibody. The financial support of Telethon-Italy (grant no. GGP030248) is also gratefully acknowledged.

References

1. Di Giaimo, R., Riccio, M., Santi, S., Galeotti, C., Ambrosetti, D. C., and Melli, M. (2002) New insights into the molecular basis of progressive myoclonus epilepsy: a multiprotein complex with cystatin B. *Hum. Mol. Genet.* **11,** 2941–2950.
2. Tsien, R. Y. and Waggoner, A. (1990) Fluorophores for confocal microscopy: photophysics and photochemistry, in *Handbook of Biological Confocal Microscopy* (Pawley, J. B., ed.), Plenum, New York, pp. 153–161.
3. Wells, S. and Johnson, I. (1994) *Three-Dimensional Confocal Microscopy: Volume Investigation of Biological Systems* (Stevens, J. K. et al., eds.), Academic Press, London U.K., pp. 101–129.
4. Riccio, M., Di Giaimo, R., Pianetti, S., Palmieri, P. P., Melli, M., and Santi, S. (2001). Nuclear localization of cystatin b, the cathepsin inhibitor implicated in myoclonus epilepsy (EPM1). *Exp. Cell Res.* **262,** 84–94.
5. Spisni, E., Griffoni, C., Santi, S., Riccio, M., Marulli, R., Bartolini, G., et al. (2001) Colocalization prostacyclin (PGI2) synthase–caveolin-1 in endothelial cells and new roles for PGI2 in angiogenesis. *Exp. Cell Res.* **266,** 31–43.
6. Manders, E. M. M., Verbeek, F. J., and Aten, J. A. (1993) Measurement of co-localization of objects in dualcolor confocal images. *J. Microsc.* **169,** 375–382.
7. Tabellini, G., Bortul, R., Santi, S., Riccio, M., Baldini, G., Cappellini, A., et al. (2003) Diacylglycerol kinase-theta is localized in the speckle domains of the nucleus. *Exp. Cell Res.* **287,** 143–154.

Index